MD

# Dr Dawn ⌐ ⌐ ...Jiabetes

Dr Dawn Harper is a GP based in Gloucestershire, working at an NHS surgery in Stroud. She has been working as a media doctor for nearly ten years. Dawn is best known as one of the presenters on Channel 4's award-winning programme *Embarrassing Bodies*, which has run for seven series and two years ago celebrated its hundredth episode. Spin-offs have included *Embarrassing Fat Bodies*, *Embarrassing Teen Bodies* and *Embarrassing Bodies: Live from the clinic*.

Dawn is the presenter of Channel 4's series *Born Naughty?*, one of the doctors on ITV1's *This Morning* and the resident GP on the health hour on LBC radio. She writes for a variety of publications, including *Healthspan*, *Healthy Food Guide* and *NetDoctor*. Her first book, *Dr Dawn's Health Check*, was published by Mitchell Beazley. *Dr Dawn's Guide to Healthy Eating for Diabetes* is one of five Dr Dawn Guides published by Sheldon Press in 2016. Dawn qualified at London University in 1987. When not working, she is a keen cyclist and an enthusiastic supporter of children's charities. Her website is at <www.drdawn.com>. Follow her on Twitter @drdawnharper.

Azmina Govindji is an award-winning dietitian, international speaker and bestselling author. She is a media spokesperson for the British Dietetic Association, resident dietitian to <www.patient.co.uk>, and a regular contributor to the NHS Choices website. Her television appearances include Sky and ITV breakfast news, *This Morning* as nutritionist (2006–7), *The One Show*, *The Wright Stuff* and BBC's *Watchdog*. She is co-founder of the award-winning RDUK Twitter chats that reach an average of two million people and involve between 60 and 85 expert nutrition participants.

Azmina has written over a dozen books on weight management and diabetes, including cookbooks that are available worldwide. She was chief dietitian to Diabetes UK for eight years and now runs her own nutrition consultancy. She offers authoritative opinion on a range of diet-related topics, and her lively personality and down-to-earth approach help her to simplify scientific dietary principles into realistic hints and tips. Azmina is a mum of two who believes that healthy food can be tasty, and she's passionate about helping people make sense of the hype around diet. Her website is at <www.azminanutrition.com>. Follow her on Twitter @AzminaNutrition or find her on Facebook at Azmina Nutrition.

# Overcoming Common Problems Series

*Selected titles*

A full list of titles is available from Sheldon Press,
36 Causton Street, London SW1P 4ST and on our website at
www.sheldonpress.co.uk

# Overcoming Common Problems Series

# Overcoming Common Problems Series

Overcoming Common Problems

# Dr Dawn's Guide to Healthy Eating for Diabetes

DR DAWN HARPER

Recipes by
AZMINA GOVINDJI

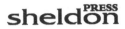
sheldon PRESS

First published in Great Britain in 2016

Sheldon Press
36 Causton Street
London SW1P 4ST
www.sheldonpress.co.uk

The authors and publisher have made every effort to ensure that the
external website and email addresses included in this book are correct and
up to date at the time of going to press. The authors and publisher are not
responsible for the content, quality or continuing accessibility of the sites.

*British Library Cataloguing-in-Publication Data*
A catalogue record for this book is available from the British Library

ISBN 978–1–84709–389–9
eBook ISBN 978–1–84709–394–3

Typeset by Fakenham Prepress Solutions, Fakenham, Norfolk NR21 8NN
First printed in Great Britain by Ashford Colour Press
Subsequently digitally reprinted in Great Britain

eBook by Fakenham Prepress Solutions, Fakenham, Norfolk NR21 8NN

Produced on paper from sustainable forests

# Contents

# Note to the reader

The dietary advice and recipes in this book are intended as a general guide, and not as a substitute for the medical advice of your doctor. Always keep to the advice of your own dietitian and doctor, particularly with respect to any symptoms that may require diagnosis or medical attention.

# Introduction

Patients often tell me I am lucky because I am obviously one of those people who is naturally slim. In fact. I'm one of the few people who knows that she isn't lucky! Through my work on Channel 4's *Embarrassing Bodies*, I have been tested for no end of things, but some of the most interesting experiences have been being tested for a whole host of fat genes – and I pretty much have a full house. I have also had my gut flora analysed. We all have about 2 kg of good bacteria in our guts that help us digest our food and they come from two main bacterial families. We have different proportions of these families. One family is significantly better at absorbing energy from our food and much work is being done looking at the possibility of altering gut flora to help with weight loss, but yes, you guessed it, I have 98 per cent of the family that are more efficient at extracting energy. So, I am actually genetically and biologically pre-programmed to be overweight. This news wasn't a huge surprise to me as I have always felt that I have gained weight more easily than my friends. I really watch what I eat and exercise regularly and I know that if I let that slip the scales tell the story.

A pound of fat is the equivalent to 3,500 calories and those of you who have tried to lose weight in the past will have been told that if you can restrict your daily calorie intake by 500 calories a day that will lead to a weight loss of a pound over the course of a week. The thing is it is much easier to overeat by 500 calories a day than it is to undereat by 500 calories a day. The average woman needs around 2,000 calories a day and the average man 2,500 calories. These are guesstimates though because bigger people may need more calories just to move those extra pounds around. and the more active you are the more you can afford to take in. If I were to eat an extra 500 calories a day every day for a year, I would gain 22.2 kg which would take my body mass index (see Chapter 2) from a healthy 20 to 29, which is bordering on clinically obese, and that would put me at significant risk of developing type 2 diabetes. The problem is, it is all too easy to eat those extra calories. In the western world we live in an obesogenic society. Food is readily available, and much of it the wrong food, portion sizes have rocketed and we are more sedentary than generations before us. In addition, 80 per cent of us don't achieve the recommended levels of 30 minutes of exercise five times a week.

There are 3.2 million people in the UK with diabetes mellitus; 90 per cent of those are people with type 2 diabetes and the reason that a lot of these people have diabetes is related to weight. On top of that, today, there could be another 750,000 people walking around with type 2 diabetes who are yet to be diagnosed. And on top of that there are an estimated 11.5 million people today who are at risk of type 2 diabetes. We spend £1 million per hour in the NHS on managing diabetes. You don't need a financial or business brain to work out that if the NHS is struggling to fund itself today (which it is), then we could be seeing the end of our NHS very soon if we don't ALL act now.

In this book I want to explain the risks associated with having diabetes and help you to do all that you can to reduce your chances of developing any of the complications. And I am delighted to have teamed up with Azmina Govindji to provide you with some diabetes-friendly recipes that all the family can enjoy.

# 1

# Diabetes – the facts

In this book when I talk about diabetes, I am referring to diabetes mellitus. Diabetes insipidus is a different condition where you have problems controlling the balance of water in your body. Like diabetes mellitus it can make you excessively thirsty, but it is not linked to a problem with the pancreas, being overweight or obese. It is due to a problem either in the brain or in the kidneys. There are two types of diabetes mellitus. Type 2 is by far the most common type, accounting for 90 to 95 per cent of all adults with diabetes, and is largely related to excess weight. Type 1 diabetes is not linked to weight. It is a condition where your body develops antibodies to the beta cells in your pancreas. These are the cells that produce insulin and very quickly your insulin levels drop.

## Type 1 diabetes

Type 1 diabetes usually appears in younger people and often in children.

### What causes type 1 diabetes?

Type 1 diabetes is a disorder of the immune system, where the body produces antibodies to its own pancreas and stops the production of insulin. We are not sure why this happens but researchers are looking into the possibility that it is triggered by a virus in those that are susceptible. There is also a genetic component of type 1 diabetes in that it does seem to run in families.

### What are the symptoms of type 1 diabetes?

The most common symptoms are feeling excessively thirsty and passing more urine. You may also feel very tired and lethargic and tend to lose weight unexpectedly. You may notice that you get recurrent infections, particularly recurrent thrush, and that any wounds are slow to heal. There can also be blurred vision as the lens of the eye changes shape. If left undiagnosed, meaning that your blood sugar levels are allowed to run very high, you may vomit and develop fruity smelling breath. This is a medical emergency and may also be associated with abdominal pain. If sugar levels are allowed to continue to rise unchecked, this can ultimately cause a fit or coma so don't delay.

## How is type 1 diabetes diagnosed?

A simple blood test will show if your sugar levels are high: if your blood sugar is greater than 11.1 mmol/litre then a diagnosis is made straight away. Type 1 diabetes is also diagnosed if the blood sugar level of a fasting blood sample is greater than 7 mmol/litre. If your sugar level is high but not this high, you will be asked to do something called a glucose tolerance test (GTT; see below). Another blood test, called the glycated haemoglobin (HbA1c), gives us an idea of how well blood sugar levels have been controlled in recent weeks. If it is greater than 6.5 per cent this is also diagnostic of diabetes; the HbA1c test is also used to monitor diabetes after diagnosis.

## How is type 1 diabetes treated?

Type 1 diabetes is treated with insulin. Insulin can be given as individual injections and there are many different types. Some are short acting, meaning their effect doesn't last long; some injections have intermediate action; and some are long acting. You may well need a combination of different types. Insulin can also be given via a pump, which means fewer injections. If you are injecting regularly you will be advised to rotate your injection sites as repeated in injections at the same site will be uncomfortable and can cause changes in the underlying fatty tissue. These changes are called lipodystrophy and look like dimples and lumps under the skin. You will also need to follow a diet and lifestyle like the one described on pages 5–6 for people with type 2 diabetes.

# Type 2 diabetes

Type 2 diabetes used to also be called adult onset or maturity onset diabetes because it was seen in older people, generally over 40 years. These alternative names have now been dropped because that is not the case. Type 2 diabetes is usually linked to being overweight and, because we are becoming bigger as a nation and lots of young people are now clinically obese, we are seeing type 2 diabetes in young adults and even in children. Unlike type 1 diabetes, type 2 diabetes develops slowly. If it is picked up early then often it can be managed with diet alone but if left untreated will need prescription medication and ultimately some people with type 2 diabetes will need insulin by injection. Type 2 diabetes develops because either you have become resistant to the effect of insulin, so normal insulin levels just aren't enough to keep your blood sugar under control, or your body doesn't make enough insulin. In some cases it can be a mixture of both.

## Who gets type 2 diabetes?

More people than you think! It is estimated that in the UK alone while you are reading this, there are 750,000 people walking around getting on with their day to day life who have diabetes and have no idea. Because the symptoms can be vague (see below) and come on so insidiously it is perfectly possible to have the condition and not be aware that you are unwell.

Risk factors for type 2 diabetes include the following:

- *Weight* Being clinically overweight (BMI 25–30; or above 23 for people of Asian descent) or clinically obese (BMI >30) significantly increases your risk and most people with type 2 diabetes are overweight.
- *Waist circumference* Women with waist circumferences of greater than 80 cm (31.5 inches) and greater than 94 cm (37 inches) for men; or 90 cm (35.5 inches) if you are an Asian or Afro-Caribbean male.
- *Ethnicity* Type 2 diabetes is about five times more common in people of Asian and Afro-Caribbean descent.
- *Family history* If your mother, father, brother, sister or child has diabetes, you are more likely to develop the condition.

- *Impaired glucose tolerance* If it is found, on routine testing, that you have a slightly raised glucose level which is not high enough to make a diagnosis of diabetes but is higher than normal, you will be asked to have what is called a glucose tolerance test. This involves having nothing to eat or drink for 8 or 12 hours. You will have a blood test, which is referred to as the 'fasting sample'. You will then be given a sugary drink containing a known amount of glucose and blood samples are taken again at given intervals to see how your body manages that known amount of sugar. If your body struggles to get your blood sugar level back to the normal range then this is called impaired glucose tolerance and puts you at increased risk of developing type 2 diabetes.
- *Pregnancy* If you have impaired glucose tolerance or develop diabetes during pregnancy this usually resolves after the baby is born, but it does increase your risk of developing type 2 diabetes later in life.

## How is type 2 diabetes diagnosed?

The symptoms of type 2 diabetes are vague and come on slowly. You may experience lethargy and increased thirst. You may find that you are passing urine more frequently and you may have recurrent infections, such as thrush, but because they develop slowly over many, many months a lot of people don't really notice so most cases of type 2 diabetes are picked up after routine health checks. In the first instance your doctor may notice there is sugar in your urine, which is picked up on urine dip-stick testing. If this is found you will be asked to have a blood test, usually on a fasting sample. That means having nothing to eat or drink for several hours (usually about eight hours, so in most instances this would mean overnight) before your blood test. Fasting blood sugar levels should be between 3.6  and 6.1 mmol/litre. If fasting sugar levels are higher than 7 mmol/litre, or if what we call a random glucose level, i.e. one taken at any time of the day, is greater than 11.1 mmol/litre this is diagnostic of diabetes. If an individual has no symptoms but the abnormality is picked up on routine testing then we repeat the tests to confirm the diagnosis but one test is enough for diagnosis if a person has symptoms of type 2 diabetes.

## How is type 2 diabetes managed?

In the first instance you will probably be asked to have an appointment with the practice nurse to talk through what you can do to change your diet and lifestyle. For some, lifestyle changes alone may be all that is needed and I will go into this in more depth later on – it is important that you know exactly what you can and can't eat. It may feel daunting at first but once you have read this book hopefully you will have a clearer idea of what you need to do. While you are waiting for your first appointment with the practice nurse, try to keep a food diary so that the nurse (and you!) can see where you might be going wrong and give you some tips on how you manage your eating habits in the future. You will need to adopt a low-fat, -salt and -sugar diet. Low fat, because managing your weight is crucial; low salt, because people with diabetes are prone to high blood pressure and kidney problems; and low sugar, because by definition, people with diabetes have difficulty handling and processing sugar and, of course, low sugar will help keep your weight under control too. As a rough guide, your diet should look like this:

- total fat less than 35 per cent of total calorie intake;
- trans fats and saturated fats should constitute less than 33 per cent of total fat intake;
- total carbohydrates should make up 40–60 per cent of your total calorie intake.

It's tough but you can reduce your fat intake by limiting fried or processed foods and high-fat snacks, such as crisps, cake and biscuits; you will also need to be careful with sugar intake from fizzy drinks, squashes and cordials and limit cakes and biscuits. You should choose foods with a low glycaemic index, which means foods that produce less of a peak in blood sugar levels. So, for example, the blood sugar peak seen after eating pasta is much lower than that after eating chips because pasta has a lower glycaemic index than potato.

Not everyone with type 2 diabetes is overweight but the majority are, and tackling your weight will be a priority for you. It is likely to be a long haul but even modest weight loss can make a real difference. Depending on the blood results, your GP and nurse may suggest that you look at lifestyle changes alone for a few months. If they can see your HbA1c returning to normal as a result of these changes then you may not need to do anything more other than stick to your new healthy living plan.

## What if my blood tests remain abnormal?

If your blood tests remain abnormal despite making changes to your lifestyle, your doctor will prescribe medication to help bring your blood sugar levels under control. It is important that you persevere with lifestyle changes, as even if you need medication now, as you continue to bring your weight down and improve your fitness you may find that you will be able to come off your medication. Although please don't ever be tempted to try this without the help of your doctor. There are several types of tablets used to keep blood sugar levels under control.

**Metformin** The drug metformin is a biguanide. It works by enhancing the use of available glucose. It is the first drug we use in type 2 diabetes that is associated with weight issues and, since most, although not all, people with type 2 diabetes are overweight, this is often the first drug of choice. It improves sensitivity to insulin and may help with weight loss.

**Sulfonylureas** These drugs work by enhancing insulin secretion, so by definition they are only useful if the pancreas is capable of producing some insulin. There are different sulfonylureas and which one you are prescribed will depend on your individual circumstances. They have different lengths of action, that is, depending on which type you have, each dose you take works for a different length of time – some of the more long-acting types may mean that you are at risk of becoming hypoglycaemic; this is when your blood sugar falls too low. This can be a medical emergency, so your doctor will fine tune which particular sulfonylurea is best for you. The sulfonylureas include glibenclamide, gliclazide, glimepiride, glipizide and tolbutamide.

**Nateglinide and repaglinide** These drugs stimulate the release of insulin. They work very quickly after being taken, but they don't last for long so they are taken immediately before eating. Nateglinide is only licensed to be used in conjunction with metformin, but repaglinide can be used on its own in people with type 2 diabetes who are not overweight or who cannot tolerate metformin.

**Pioglitazone** This drug works by reducing insulin resistance. It can be used on its own or alongside metformin or a sulfonylurea but it must be used with care. It has been shown to increase the risk of heart failure when combined with insulin, so shouldn't be used in anyone with known heart failure, and all patients who take this drug need to be closely monitored.

**Gliptins** These drugs increase insulin secretion and reduce glucagon secretion. Glucagon is another pancreatic hormone which works to raise blood sugar levels when they start to fall. They can be used on their own or in conjunction with metformin or a sulfonylurea, or with pioglitazone. They include saxagliptin, sitagliptin and vildagliptin.

**Acarbose** This drug delays the digestion and absorption of carbohydrate and sugar from the gut. It is generally reserved for those patients who cannot tolerate other anti-diabetic medication.

### What if tablets can't control my type 2 diabetes?

If you have tried lifestyle changes and despite adding in tablets your sugar levels and HbA1c levels remain abnormal, your doctor will suggest you try injection therapy. There are two main types of injection therapy:

- *insulin,* see type 1 diabetes;
- *exenatide and liraglutide,* these drugs increase insulin secretion, reduce glucagon secretion and delay gastric emptying so that there is a slower delivery of food to the small intestine where the sugar is absorbed.

## Will I need other medication?

If you have diabetes, whether it is type 1 or type 2, your risk of developing high blood pressure, high cholesterol and heart disease, among other things, increases. Your doctor will want to monitor you for these problems and will advise on whether you need medication. The good news through all of this, though, is that if you persevere with your lifestyle changes you could potentially, under the supervision of your medical team, come off all the medicines. That is quite some incentive!

## How will my diabetes be monitored?

You will need regular review at your GP surgery and maybe also at the hospital. You will need blood tests to check your glucose levels and your HbA1c; you will also need cholesterol blood tests and tests to check your kidney function. You will have your eyes checked every year, as diabetes can affect your vision, and you will have regular blood pressure checks and checks on your sensation and your feet. It is important that whenever you have an appointment you leave knowing when the next one will be and whether it is down to you to make a note of when to go back or you will be informed near the appointment date.

## Why is it so important to control my sugar level when I don't feel unwell with it?

You may feel totally well with higher than normal blood sugar levels but persistently high glucose levels in the blood damages the blood vessels, the body's organs and the nerves. In real terms, this means that if you ignore your condition you are at significant risk of some serious health issues in the future. I will cover each of these in depth in this book but briefly they include:

- heart disease
- stroke
- high blood pressure
- high cholesterol
- visual problems

- kidney disease
- nerve damage
- foot problems
- sexual problems
- problems in pregnancy.

# 2

# Managing your weight

## Getting started

If you have recently been diagnosed with type 2 diabetes, your doctor will have weighed and measured you to know your waist measurement and calculate your body mass index (BMI). Women with waist circumferences of greater than 80 cm (31.5 inches) and men with waists greater than 94 cm (37 inches), or 90 cm (35.5 inches) for Asian or Afro-Caribbean males, are at greater risk of type 2 diabetes. Your BMI is your weight, in kilogrammes, divided by the square of your height, in metres:

BMI = weight in kgs divided by (height in metres times height in metres)

You should aim for a BMI of between 18.5 and 25 (or 23 if you are of Asian descent). If you have type 2 diabetes and are overweight, you may be champing at the bit to get started on your new healthy living regime, but to give yourself the best chance of success you may need to spend a little time identifying your weaknesses. We all have them and there is nothing wrong with that; we just need to know how to deal with them. I am lucky in many ways. I don't have a sweet tooth so for me I can live with chocolate and biscuits in the cupboard for weeks without being tempted. That's not because I have more will power than the next person. It is just because they don't appeal. But pass me a plate of cheese and then I struggle not to eat it all. It took me a long while to recognize this in myself but, now that I know, I try to avoid buying cheese for a while when I am trying to get myself back in check; for example, after a holiday or the Christmas break when most of us overindulge.

Your weaknesses may be glaringly obvious to you, but they may not be. It really is worth spending a couple of weeks before you start your new healthy living regime just documenting what you eat, when and why. And I mean everything. So if it is polishing off the spare chips from the kids' plates as you were clearing the table, you need to write it down – and try to think about why you ate them. Was it because you were hungry and the temptation was just too much? Was it just because they were there and you had eaten them before you even really had time to think about it? This is important because the most difficult part of your new regime will be not cheating.

We all lead busy lives and it is amazing how easy it is to overeat especially with snacks. If you are really honest with yourself during your two-week diary keeping, you will very quickly be able to see your weak points. It is hard, I know, because as soon as you start to document things, it is human nature to start to alter what you do because by definition you are thinking about it. Hopefully, at the end of your fortnight you will have a very clear record of your eating habits. There will be things that you knew all along but other parts will surprise you. If you go for second helpings try to make a note of how long you left it before you were reaching for the serving spoon and were you having more because it was just so tasty or were you still feeling hungry.

So now you have the facts in front of you and you will have identified your weaknesses and we are almost ready to get started. Whatever your weak points are, we need to make a plan as to how we deal with them. So let's just say it is chocolate biscuits. First of all ask yourself if you really need them in the house? Of course, if you live with others then it is unfair to ask them to go without unless they are really behind you on this new journey and are happy to do so. If you have to have them in the house are there some brands which are less tempting than others? Could you substitute those? Why do you buy them? Are they just too irresistible when you are doing the shopping? Can you force yourself not to go down that aisle? Are there times when you feel stronger than others? Could you time your weekly shop to be done when your willpower seems to be stronger? Have you considered internet shopping? If you really have to have them in the house, try leaving yourself a note on the biscuit tin. Nothing nasty but maybe something along the lines of 'Do you really want this? If you do you can have one if you still feel the same way in 5 minutes'. You would be amazed how often you will find your willpower in just a few minutes, and you will be able to keep to your healthy eating plan. Alternatively, perhaps keep a couple of biscuits in a separate tin so if you get that 'I'm stressed so I'll eat all the biscuits' thing, there are only two biscuits to eat!

I had one lovely patient on *Embarrassing Fat Bodies* who had worked incredibly hard and lost 8 stone. She had so much to be proud of. She did it on her own with a healthy-eating and regular-exercise plan. It took her months but, believe me, she was unrecognizable physically and emotionally. Her light-bulb moment had been collecting a set of holiday snaps from the chemist. The first photograph was one of her sitting on a boat in the Mediterranean. She was a big girl and she said when she saw that photograph she saw herself as others saw her and she became very upset. We have long accepted that anorexics see a different image in the mirror than we do – they see fat bits that simply aren't there – and I believe this lady saw a different image in the mirror. She knew she was buying size 26 clothes but in her mind she had kidded herself that she was a size 18 and she was comfortable with that. That photograph forced her to take her head out of the sand and accept that she was unhealthily overweight. She hated that picture, but she used it to advantage. She cut it down and kept it in the front of her purse. She told me that every time she thought she wanted a burger, or a binge on chocolate, she had to get past that photograph to get to her money and nine times out of ten that image was enough to help her decide against her moment of weakness. She had a strategy that most of the time kept her on track and worked for her. It may be something totally different for you – it may be that a photograph of you looking slim will motivate you – but, with a bit of thought, you will be able to formulate a plan that will help you in moments of weakness.

## Healthy eating for diabetes

The whole ethos of changing your diet to help manage your diabetes is about making small but sustainable changes – so don't panic. I have always been a firm believer that there is no such thing as a bad food, just plenty of bad diets. Even as someone with diabetes you can have the occasional chocolate or crisp as treats, but incorporate them into your diet every day and you are going to run in to more trouble with your diabetes! When my children were small I used to have what I called the 'treats cupboard' where I kept biscuits and cake. As they got older and could open the cupboard and help themselves we laughed that if a treat was a treat, it had to be just that – something special that you indulge in occasionally and not part of everyday life!

In the modern-day western world we have rather lost sight of what is a healthy balanced diet, so don't beat yourself up. We live in an obesogenic society where food (and often the wrong food) is plentiful and we are all more sedentary than we were. I know my children spend more time sitting in front of some sort of screen than I ever did. They are active kids but with the availability of laptops, tablets, games consoles and 24-hour television, it is so easy to spend much of our waking day sitting down, which means is that if we don't make conscious decisions to deal with our lifestyles we are going to be fighting an uphill battle with our weight.

So what is healthy eating? It is about getting the right balance of all the food groups and in the right proportions (Figure 1).

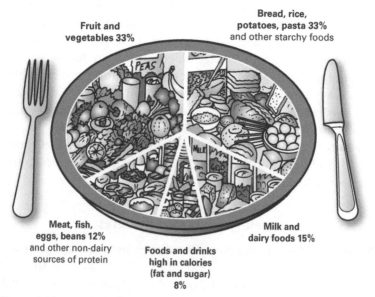

**Figure 1 The eatwell plate**
This plate model is due to be revised by the UK Department of Health in the near future.

## Starchy foods

Starchy foods contain carbohydrate, which is an essential source of energy in our diet. Many diets recommend cutting out carbohydrates or keeping your intake to a minimum. We are back to the 'no such thing as a bad food, just a bad diet' argument here. Carbohydrates are not bad for you, but in excess the body will lay down the extra calories as fat stores for leaner times and, to be honest, it's not so much the food itself as the way it is cooked. Let's look at potatoes – a great source of starch but if you deep fry them in fat then you are loading on the calories. Starchy foods should constitute about a third to a half of your total daily calorie intake and include bread, potatoes, pasta and rice. As a general rule, wholegrain varieties are better than refined grains. At least half of the grains you eat should be whole grains and, to be honest, the greater the proportion the better. Wholegrain simply means that the bran hasn't been removed by milling so it is higher in fibre; this includes brown rice and pasta, and brown bread. Refined grains are milled, which strips out the bran, and these include white bread, white rice and white pasta. It can be difficult to tell though as some 'brown bread' may be brown because of colouring so get into the habit of looking at food labels and look for the word *whole*.

## Fruit and vegetables

It's good to know that the five portions of fruit and vegetables message is getting out there. There has been much debate about whether this recommendation should be increased but, for me, if I could ensure that we all achieved our *five a day*, then I think we would be getting somewhere! Fruit and vegetables should account for about a third of your daily calorie intake. There is still a lot of confusion as to what constitutes a portion, and remember frozen, canned and dried fruit and vegetables all count. Actually, fresh fruit juice also counts but only as one portion, irrespective of how much you drink, and that is because much of the fibre is removed during the process of juicing; the importance of fruit and vegetables in your diet is because they contain vitamins, minerals and some carbohydrate, mainly in the form of sugar, but also fibre. I will discuss what constitutes a portion in a later section.

## Meat, fish and other protein

Protein is an essential part of our diet. We need it to repair tissues and build muscle. Protein-rich foods are also a good source of vitamin B12, which is vital to maintain a healthy nervous system and make new red blood cells. These foods also tend to be a good source of iron, zinc and magnesium. Try to eat at least two portions of oily fish a week. This means mackerel, sardines, trout or salmon as they are rich in omega-3 oils, which help prevent against heart disease and, as an added benefit, will keep your skin and bones healthy.

## Fat

Fat is the most energy-dense food which is why overindulging with fat will predispose to weight gain and most of us probably eat too much saturated fat, which is the fat found in butter, cheese, pastries, cakes and biscuits. Saturated fats and trans fats will not only predispose you to weight gain but can also raise cholesterol levels and increase the risk of heart disease. As someone with diabetes your risk of developing these conditions is already raised so your fat intake should be no more than a third of your total calorie intake and, of this, only a third should be saturated or trans fats. It's a case of getting into the habit of checking food labels. This will seem very time consuming at first but you will be amazed at how quickly you get used to knowing what you are looking for. Simple things like swapping butter for olive oil (rich in unsaturated fat) will make a significant difference.

## Sugar

Adults should have no more than 25 g, or 6 teaspoons, of sugar a day. Most of us eat too much sugar and when you start analysing your diet you may be shocked at just how much sugar you are consuming. Beware 'low-fat' foods. Very often the fat is substituted with sugar to enhance the flavour so you may think you are choosing a healthy option only to find your sugar intake is too high. Most soft drinks are also laden with sugar – you would be surprised by how much you can reduce your daily calorific intake simply by swapping canned drinks for water.

## Salt

We have got used to a high-salt diet. Too much salt increases the risk of developing high blood pressure, which in turn increases the risk of heart attacks and strokes. All these conditions are more common in people with diabetes, so do look at your salt intake. You should limit your daily intake to 6 grams and, when you start looking at the hidden salt in processed foods, you will be shocked by the amounts. Try to avoid high salt-content foods and try not to add salt to food. At first this will taste bland but human taste buds adapt very quickly and within a couple of weeks you will wonder how you managed to eat such salty food!

## Alcohol

Alcohol is laden with sugar and what I call *empty calories* – calories with no nutritional benefit. But we have to be realistic. Just because you are diabetic, doesn't mean you have to be teetotal, but it does mean you should really try to stick to recommended limits. Recommended limits for alcohol are just 14 units a week for women and 21 for men and, I'm afraid I am going to frighten you now, that is significantly less than you think. We used to refer to a unit as a small glass of wine, half a pint of beer or a single measure of spirit but as beers and wines have become stronger we need to rethink this. The simple way to calculate your alcohol intake is by looking at the percentage alcohol in the drink you are drinking. The percentage alcohol shows you the number of units in a litre of that drink; so, for wine, a 75 cl bottle is three-quarters of a litre (75 cl = 750 ml; 1 litre = 1000 ml), so if the wine contains 12 per cent alcohol, the number of units in the bottle is three-quarters of 12 = 9 units. If you are pouring a glass at home it is likely to be a 250 ml glass and that will contain 3 units not 1. So beware of alcohol. It is laden with hidden calories and will play havoc with your willpower!

## Calorie comparisons

As a rough guide, carbohydrates and proteins contain about 4 calories per gram, alcohol contains 7 calories per gram and fat contains 9 calories per gram.

## What is a portion?

Portion size is probably one of the biggest problems in the western diet. We have simply got used to overeating. You only have to look at the size of a Mars Bar – I am sure they have doubled in size since I was a kid and, of course, what that says to us, in a subliminal way, is that that large bar of chocolate is a totally appropriate amount to eat in one go on your own. It's not!

The best way to regulate your portions is to invest in scales and jugs and spoons but we have to be practical here and you are not going to be able to carry them with you wherever you go. If you get into the habit of measuring food at home though, you will soon learn to recognize what you think should be a portion. It is also worth investing in smaller plates, bowls and wine glasses. We know that we eat up to as much as 50 per cent more from larger plates and sticking to smaller wine glasses will help you regulate your alcohol intake.

If you don't have measuring devices to hand here is rough guide to what portions should be:

- your palm is the size of a portion of meat or fish (approximately 150 grams);
- your cupped hand is the size of a portion of pasta or rice (about half a cup);
- both cupped hands is the size of a portion of salad (about one cup);
- your index finger is the size of a portion of cheese (about one tablespoon);
- your thumb is the size of a portion of jam (about one teaspoon).

## What about second helpings?

There is nothing wrong with second helpings if you really need them, but try this little experiment. Put all the food you are going to eat in a single meal on your table and sit down to eat. Actually promising yourself that you will only eat sitting down is a good habit to get into. It means you are less likely to graze on canapés, nuts and crisps. You won't clear your little boy's plate of leftovers on your way to the bin, and you won't be able to cheat on portion size. You are also likely to eat more slowly, giving your brain a chance to register that your stomach is full. If when you have finished your plate, you still want more, promise yourself you can have it if you still want it in 15 minutes. It can take a while for the hormones released from our gut to tell our brains that we are full so give them a chance and more often than not you will start to feel full and decide against that second helping.

---

### Dr Dawn's top ten tips for slimmer eating

1 Identify your weaknesses.
2 Don't buy foods that will lead you astray.
3 Buy smaller plates, bowls and glasses.
4 Put all your food on your plate before you start eating.
5 Reduce your portion size by a third.
6 Sit down to eat.
7 Eat slowly.
8 Only go back for second helpings if you have allowed your first serving to digest for 15 minutes.
9 Keep healthy snacks with you to combat hunger pangs.
10 Drink more water.

---

## Exercise for managing diabetes

There is no doubt that the best way to lose weight and to keep it off is to combine a healthy-eating programme with regular exercise, but you need to pick your exercise. Many gym memberships are paid for by well-intentioned people who part with their hard-earned cash, but give up going after a few weeks. Sadly, just paying your monthly subscription isn't going to be enough. You have to go and go regularly! So now is another time to have a think and be honest with yourself. If you hate the gym, it doesn't matter how smart the facilities look, you may force yourself to stick with exercising there for a small number of weeks, maybe even a small number of months but, as sure as eggs are eggs, you won't be doing it this time next year. And exercise is like healthy eating. If you have diabetes, you need to make small changes that, hand on heart, you think you will be able to keep up for good. I know this because, over the years, I have joined gyms. I join in January and, by spring, I have usually fallen by the wayside – and that's because I get bored in a gym.

A few years ago I was run over by a car and shattered my left knee. Part of my rehabilitation was sitting on a static bicycle in a physiotherapy gym, trying to flex my knee enough to do a single revolution. When I achieved this, I was so desperate to build the strength up in my damaged leg and regain full mobility, that I started cycling in the lanes near my house. I found that this was something I really enjoyed. Ten minutes on a bike in the gym and I'm clock watching but cycling in the countryside just ticked boxes for me and I started cycling with friends in the village. I have always been a great believer in exercising with friends because when your motivation is low they will spur you on, and you will do the same for them. Before I knew it, I had signed up to a charity ride from London to Paris – and that ticked another box. There is nothing like the fear of failure to make sure you get out and train whatever you motivation or the weather outside. So I learned a lot about myself: I prefer exercising outside; I need friends to force me out when I'm feeling lazy; and I need a challenge to make me stick to my training schedule. The boxes you need to tick may be completely different for you and they may not be obvious to begin with but as you start your new healthy living regime, it is worth giving this some thought. Maybe you love dancing? A dance class is a great way to exercise. Perhaps you could help a friend walk their dog? Maybe it should be something as simple as walking with a work colleague at lunchtimes?

## Keeping active and doing regular exercise

Anything we can do to keep moving will burn calories. We recommend that everyone walks at least 10,000 paces a day and, ideally, that should be your baseline with formal exercise on top of that but – again – be realistic about your goals. If you have been something of a couch potato in recent years, then just achieving 10,000 steps a day will be a major achievement. And it can be surprisingly difficult to do. The average pace is 50–75 cm long which means, if you achieve your 10,000 steps, you will walk 5–7.5 km in a day just going about your business! A while back I decided to practise what I preach and invested in a pedometer. I think of myself as quite an active person and certainly at weekends I had no problem clocking in my 10,000 paces. Busy days in surgery were a totally different matter, and I found that sitting at my desk calling in patients meant it was easy to get to 6.30 p.m. and be frighteningly short of my target. I decided then to get up and walk to the waiting room rather than use an intercom calling system. It meant I could maintain my activity levels on my surgery days when I was pretty sedentary and I actually prefer it. It is so much more personal than calling people through using a tannoy. This simple change meant I was staying on target and, in this day of internet technology, emails, texts and all the other ways of communicating with the outside world without actually moving, it can be all too easy to get to the end of your day without having moved much at all.

It doesn't matter what you do, but if your job is sedentary you will have to make a definite decision to move more. Maybe you get off the bus or the tube a stop early? Maybe you use the stairs instead of an escalator or a lift? Maybe you promise yourself that you will walk over to your colleague's desk to discuss an issue rather than just press 'send' on an email? Whatever you decide to do, invest in a pedometer and start counting your daily steps. This is what I call baseline activity. Once you have achieved this, you need to think about exercise on top and, ideally, you should be aiming for 30 minutes a day, or at least five times a week. It doesn't matter what it is but you need to get a bit short of breath doing it. The sort of shortness of breath that means you talk in short phrases and need to catch your breath. If you are gasping for air you are overdoing it and need to take the pressure off, but if you are chatting happily then don't kid yourself – you may be keeping active but you are not truly exercising in my book and you need to push yourself a bit harder!

If you want to get a little more technical, buy yourself a heart rate monitor to wear while you are exercising. When you are fit, you should aim for a pulse rate between 70 and 85 per cent of your maximum heart rate (MHR). If you are just starting out 60 per cent of your MHR is probably more realistic. You can calculate your MHR by subtracting your age from 220 if you are a man, or 210 if you are a woman. So, if you are a man aged 40, your MHR is:

$$220 - 40 = 180.$$

Your optimum training range is 70–85 per cent of 180, which is:

70% of 180 = (70 ÷ 100) × 180 = 126 beats per minute
85% of 180 = (85 ÷ 100) × 180 = 153 beats per minute.

The great thing about exercise is that it burns calories – but it also does so much more. If you exercise regularly, you will boost your metabolism. What this means, in real terms, is that you will burn more calories just sitting at your desk than an identical person who hadn't done the exercise.

# 3

# Heart disease

As someone with type 2 diabetes, you are at an increased risk of developing heart disease so in this chapter I will discuss exactly what we mean by heart disease and what you can do to minimize the effects of any other risk factors you may have. Coronary heart disease (CHD) means that there is reduced blood supply to the heart muscle, usually because the coronary arteries are getting furred up. It can present as a heart attack or as angina.

## What is a heart attack?

A heart attack is where the blood supply to part of the heart is cut off causing the muscle supplied by that vessel to die. A heart attack is also sometimes called a myocardial infarction (MI) – myocardial meaning heart muscle and infarction meaning dead tissue. A heart attack, or MI, usually presents with a central crushing chest pain, which may radiate into the left arm, neck or jaw. Sometimes the pain is felt in both arms and sometimes there is no pain but the attack is picked up on an ECG tracing. The pain may be associated with shortness of breath, feeling sick or light headed. You may feel clammy and those around you may think you look pale or grey. This is a medical emergency and you or someone near you should call 999 immediately.

The most common cause of a heart attack is a clot blocking an artery. The size and severity of the heart attack depends on the size of the blood vessel that is blocked. If a small artery is blocked then a small area of muscle will be affected and you are less likely to have long-term problems. If one of the main coronary arteries is blocked then a large part of muscle is affected and unless the blood vessel can be opened again quickly, you are likely to be left very short of breath on minimal exertion because the heart simply can't pump hard enough with the healthy muscle that is left.

## Who gets heart attacks?

There are a number of risk factors for heart attacks. Some we can do nothing about. These include:

- *age*, most heart attacks occur in the over 50s;
- *gender*, men are more at risk than premenopausal women as oestrogen protects the heart, but after the menopause the risk for women starts to increase;
- *ethnicity*, Asian and Afro-Caribbean people are more at risk than Caucasians;
- *family history*, if your father or brother had coronary heart disease or a thrombotic stroke (a stroke caused by a blood clot) before the age of 55 or your mother or sister before the age of 60, this increases your risk.

Other risk factors are down to lifestyles and as someone with diabetes these are the things that you can and must do something about.

**Smoking** The more you smoke, the greater the risk. In fact it is thought that 20 per cent of deaths from coronary artery disease in men and 17 per cent in women are due to smoking, but the good news is that you can reduce your risk by 25 per cent if you stop smoking and once you have given up for 10 years, your risks return to that of a non-smoker!

**Obesity** It is thought that as many as a third of all CHD deaths are due to poor diet. The risk is highest when the excess weight is carried around the middle. If you took two identical women, same height and same weight but one woman carries her weight around her middle (apple shaped) and the other carries her weight around her hips and thighs (pear shaped), the apple would have a greater risk of developing heart disease than the pear.

**Lack of exercise** You should aim to exercise for at least 30 minutes at least 5 times a week.

**Hypertension** See Chapter 5.

**Cholesterol** See Chapter 6. Cholesterol is implicated in nearly half of all cardiac deaths.

**Alcohol** Consistently drinking more than the recommended 14 units per week for women or 21 units per week for men increases your risk of coronary heart disease and binge drinking is thought to be the most risky.

### How is a heart attack diagnosed?

A doctor will immediately suspect a heart attack in anyone presenting with the symptoms mentioned above and will arrange an ECG. There are specific changes on the ECG tracing that occur when heart muscle is being damaged. Where those changes occur depends on which bit of muscle is being damaged. If a myocardial infarction is suspected, a blood test will be arranged looking for a rise in a chemical called troponin. When heart muscle is damaged it releases this chemical into the bloodstream and troponin levels will start to rise within 3 hours of a heart attack. They peak between 24 and 48 hours and will then return to normal over the next 5 to 14 days.

### How is a heart attack treated?

If you have a heart attack you will be probably be given an aspirin to thin your blood. You may also be offered other blood thinning agents. If doctors can restore blood flow to the heart muscle quickly (within a few hours), the damage to the heart muscle can be minimized. If your symptoms are caught early, and the facilities are available, you may be offered an injection of a clot-busting drug. You can only have this once in your lifetime as your body develops antibodies to it, so if you have had a previous heart attack where this was administered, you will not be offered it again but you may be offered an angioplasty. This is where a small wire with a balloon on the end is inserted into the large artery in your groin or arm and then, under X-ray control, is passed into the coronary artery. When it reaches the site of the blockage, the balloon can be inflated to open up the artery again. The doctors may leave a stent in the artery to keep it open.

After a heart attack you will be admitted to hospital where you will probably be looked after in a coronary care unit where the nurses and doctors have special expertise in looking after people with heart problems. You will be attached to a heart monitor so they can monitor your heart rhythm and you will have regular blood tests. Over the next few days you are likely to be started on a combination of drugs and these may include:

- *nitrates*, these drugs dilate blood vessels and help maintain a healthy blood flow to the heart;
- *beta blockers*, these are a group of drugs that slow the heart rate and keep a steady rhythm;
- *ACE (angiotensin converting enzyme inhibitors) inhibitors*, these lower blood pressure;
- *statins*, to lower cholesterol.

## What happens after I leave hospital?

When you leave hospital the hospital doctors will contact your GP so that he or she knows what has happened and that you are now on a new cocktail of medicines to protect your heart. You will be given a short course of drugs to take home with you (usually enough for just a couple of weeks) and then you will have to see your own GP for repeat prescriptions. You will be seen again in the hospital and they will ask you to exercise on a treadmill while monitoring your heart to see what effect any damage may have had on your exercise tolerance and you will probably be offered a cardiac rehabilitation programme where you will be able to ask questions about your personal recovery and will be told what to expect.

## What are the complications of a heart attack?

The larger the heart attack and the longer before medical help was given, the greater the risk of complications, so if you had a small heart attack which was recognized quickly and treatment given, the chances are you will make a full recovery. Larger heart attacks, especially if treatment was delayed for any reason, are more likely to develop complications and these include:

- *heart failure*, this is where the muscle is so damaged that the heart is no longer able to pump blood as effectively leading to shortness of breath, sometimes on minimal exertion, and swollen ankles;

- *rhythm problems*, these are most likely to occur in the first few hours or days after a heart attack which is why your team will keep you in hospital under surveillance.

Once you have had one heart attack you are at increased risk of another at some point in the future so it is vital that you address any lifestyle issues that put you at risk.

### What is acute coronary syndrome?

You may hear this term during your stay in hospital and it is the term used to describe a range of conditions from heart attacks that are associated with changes on the ECG, which usually means complete blockage of an artery, heart attacks that have no change in the ECG and are probably due to partial blockage of the artery, and angina.

### What is angina?

Angina usually occurs when the coronary arteries are narrowed by plaques. There is no total blockage but because the arteries are narrower, the heart muscle can't get as much blood. When you are exercising or even after eating a meal, your heart would normally pump more strongly to divert blood to the large muscles needed for exercise or to the gut to aid digestion. If the blood supply is compromised then the heart muscle struggles and this presents as a pain across the chest like that of a heart attack but it should wear off if you rest. If you are diagnosed with angina, your GP will discuss all the risk factors with you – these are the same as the ones for coronary heart disease and you will be encouraged to address these. He will start you on medication to reduce your risk of heart attack and will give you a nitrate spray which you can spray under your tongue at the onset of an attack of angina. This is rapidly absorbed into the bloodstream and will dilate the blood vessels. If angina lasts for more than 10 minutes, you should call an ambulance in case it is a heart attack. Angina can also less commonly be caused by spasm in the coronary artery walls. Angina can be described as stable when it is predictable. If you know that you are OK to walk around a supermarket but if you were to run for a bus then you would develop pain, this is stable angina. If, however, the pain is triggered by less and less exertion or even occurs while at rest, this is called unstable angina and should be considered a medical emergency as it could herald a heart attack.

## Can I drive after a heart attack?

You should not drive for at least four weeks after a heart attack. If your recovery is going well you should be fine to drive again at this stage, but if you have had complications your doctors will advise you about when you should start driving again. If you have stable angina, you are safe to drive, but if you develop pains while driving you should stop immediately and if your angina becomes unstable you must stop driving until your symptoms are back under control.

# 4

# Stroke and transient ischaemic attack

## Stroke

A stroke occurs when the blood supply to the brain is cut off. Often this is due to a blood clot forming in an area of narrowed artery usually due to atherosclerosis. Our arteries harden as we age and people with diabetes are more prone to this, but that doesn't mean a stroke is an inevitable consequence of diabetes. What it does mean is that you, more than your non-diabetic friends and relatives, will need to address any lifestyle factors that will also increase your risk. Given that there are over 150,000 strokes every year in the UK and that stroke is the most common cause of adult disability world-wide, this is something you need to take very seriously. My own late grandmother suffered a stroke and it was so sad to see such a vibrant woman become so incapacitated and dependent on others.

### What causes a stroke?

In eight out of ten cases a stroke is caused by a blood clot but sometimes it may be caused by a bleed in the brain or, rarely, by inflammation in the blood vessels supplying the brain. The way we treat a stroke varies depending on the cause and the treatment is more effective the sooner it is given, so it is vital that if you suspect a stroke you call for urgent medical help.

### How would I recognize a stroke?

Some of you may have seen the television adverts that explain what to look out for in someone having a stroke. These signs are summarised using the acronym FAST to help you remember:

- Face: there is an asymmetry of the face meaning that the person may be unable to smile on one side or have a droopy eye;

- Arm: the person may not be able to lift one arm;
- Speech may be slurred, the person may be talking gibberish or may not be able to talk at all;
- Time is of the essence. If you suspect a stroke, the sooner you can get medical help, the better the outlook. If you think this is happening to someone, call 999 immediately.

## What happens after I call 999?

If a stroke is suspected the medical team will order an urgent scan to assess whether the stroke has been caused by a bleed or a clot. If a clot is found, clot-busting drugs can be given; the more quickly these are given the more quickly the clot can be dispelled and blood supply restored to the brain. Every minute counts when dealing with a stroke so, if a clot is detected, the medical team will work hard to start this therapy as soon as possible. If you are not eligible for clot-busting drugs, you may be given aspirin or other drugs to make your blood less sticky, and if doctors notice that your heart has an abnormal rhythm, called atrial fibrillation, you will be given treatment for that to reduce your risk of further episodes. Once you have been stabilized, you will start on your rehabilitation which is likely to involve lots of different people including physiotherapists, speech therapists, occupational therapists, psychologists and of course the doctors and nurses looking after you.

## What are the long-term effects of a stroke?

About half of all stroke sufferers will be living independently six months after the event. Sadly, between 20 and 25 per cent of people who have a stroke will die. Some make a full recovery although the rehabilitation may take months but others go on to have long-term disabilities, including:

- speech difficulties
- weakness
- co-ordination and balance problems
- difficulties swallowing
- emotional lability and depression
- problems with concentration

- visual problems
- fatigue.

The speech difficulties associated with stroke may result in people having difficulty expressing themselves. The person who has had the stroke may know what they want to say but use the wrong word. They may, for example, want to know where the keys are but ask for the car. Other stroke sufferers may not be able to understand you when you talk to them because the part of the brain that processes and understands speech has been damaged, and some will be unable to speak at all. The weakness can range from a total inability to move one side of the body to varying degrees of weakness in an arm and/or leg. The visual problems mean that sometimes people will have lost the ability to see anything on one side of their visual field.

### What can I do to reduce my risks of having a stroke?

There are several changes to lifestyle that can influence your blood pressure and cholesterol level and could prevent you having a stroke. These changes are the same as those for minimizing the risk factors for heart disease (see Chapter 4).

## Transient ischaemic attack (TIA)

A transient ischaemic attack (TIA) is often referred to as a mini stroke. By this we mean, they present in exactly the same way as a stroke (remember FAST) but the symptoms recover, sometimes within minutes but always within 24 hours.

One in three people suffering a TIA will have a stroke at some point in the following year so it is important that you recognize what is happening so that you can take action to reduce that risk. One in six will have a heart attack. Reducing the risk of these events is all about doing the things that reduce your risk of a stroke generally, and taking any medication as prescribed by your doctor.

## How can you tell if you are going to be one of the unlucky ones?

The simple answer is you can't. None of us has a crystal ball but doctors use a scoring system to try to identify those most at risk. This is called the **ABCD score**:

- Age: being over 60 = 1 point;
- Blood pressure: greater than 140 mmHg systolic or 90 mmHg diastolic = 1 point;
- Clinical features: one-sided weakness = 2 points; speech difficulties = 1 point;
- Duration of symptoms: greater than one hour = 2 points; 10–59 minutes = 1 point;
- Diabetes, if present = 1 point.

A score of less than 4 is low risk, but if you score over 6 then there is significant risk of developing a stroke during the following week and it is important that you are reviewed by a specialist team with expertise in stroke management to minimize the risk of this happening.

# 5

# Hypertension

Hypertension is the medical term for high blood pressure. Blood pressure is the pressure created in the arteries as blood is pumped out of the heart. It is usually measured while sitting from the brachial artery – the artery that you can feel pulsating in the crease of your elbow. It is completely appropriate for blood pressure to be raised when we are exercising or in pain. It is also normal for blood pressure to go up when we are stressed. In evolutionary terms this was a good thing. It was a response to an adrenalin rush, which is part of the fight or flight reaction. If what is making you stressed is a looming mammoth, it's a good thing that you are wired and alert and ready to run or to stand and fight. The problem today is that our stress doesn't come in the form of an occasional mammoth. It is more likely to be produced by the daily pressures to meet deadlines, juggle family and work, and so on, so we are more likely to have high blood pressure for long periods of time.

You can feel perfectly well with high blood pressure. In fact, contrary to popular belief most people do. People with high blood pressure don't usually have headaches or blurred vision. They have no idea that they are at risk unless they are checked. As someone with diabetes, you will have regular blood pressure checks and your doctors will aim for a lower blood pressure than if you weren't diabetic. Consistently high blood pressure will put a strain on your heart. Your heart is a bit like your car engine. If you occasionally put your foot on the throttle to accelerate past a 'mammoth', your engine (heart) will cope fine. But if you spend your life with your foot on the floor (everyday stress and pressure) eventually your engine (heart) will start to show the strain.

## What is hypertension?

Blood pressure is recorded as two numbers – the systolic value is the highest pressure that system reaches and the diastolic pressure is the lowest pressure. Normal blood pressure in people without diabetes is less than 140/90 mmHg. As someone with diabetes, your doctor will aim to keep your blood pressure below 140/80 mmHg because he or she will know you are at increased risk of heart disease and stroke. If you have other complications of diabetes, such as established kidney disease for example, you doctor will be even stricter – aiming to keep your blood pressure at 130/80 or below.

About three in every ten people with type 1 diabetes will develop hypertension at some point in their lives and as many as eight out of every ten people with type 2 diabetes can expect to become hypertensive during their lifetimes.

## What can I do to lower my blood pressure?

There are several changes to lifestyle that can influence your blood pressure and these changes are the same as those for minimizing the risk factors for heart disease (see Chapter 5). It really is important that as someone with diabetes you take managing your blood pressure seriously. Just one kilo of weight loss can reduce your blood pressure by 2.5–1.5 mmHg.

## What if need medication to treat my blood pressure?

If your blood pressure remains high despite changes to your lifestyle your doctor will start you on pills. There are many different types of anti-hypertensive drugs and which ones you are prescribed will depend on your individual circumstances, what other medications you are on and what other illnesses you have. You may end up needing more than one type of pill. If you develop side effects, always discuss these with your GP as there is always an alternative, but never stop taking any prescribed medicine without talking to your doctor first. If your heart is already showing signs of strain then your GP may suggest you start a low dose of aspirin and if your cholesterol is high he or she may also give you a statin to reduce your cholesterol level. Most people who start blood pressure treatment will need to be on that treatment for life, but if you manage to lose more weight and make more changes to your lifestyle, it is possible to come off medication altogether, under supervision.

# 6

## Cholesterol

Cholesterol is a fat or lipid, which is partly made in cells in our body and partly derived from the food that we eat. Contrary to popular belief, not all cholesterol is bad and, in fact, we need some cholesterol to stay healthy. When we measure cholesterol, we measure the total cholesterol, but we also look at the levels of different lipoproteins that circulate in the bloodstream. As the name suggests these are compounds which are a combination of protein and lipid. This is the way cholesterol is transported in the bloodstream. There are several different lipoproteins but the ones particularly relevant to cholesterol are low density lipoproteins (LDLs) and high density lipoproteins (HDLs). The LDLs are often referred to as 'bad' cholesterol and the HDLs as 'good' cholesterol. The LDLs comprise the majority of the cholesterol. If you have diabetes, or have already been diagnosed with heart disease, your doctor will want to reduce your total cholesterol level, but if you are at risk of developing heart disease, he or she will be more interested in the ratio of your good cholesterol to the total level.

### What is normal cholesterol?

Cholesterol is measured in the blood in mmol per litre. For most people total cholesterol should be less than 5.0 mmol per litre, LDL cholesterol should be less than 3 mmol per litre and HDL cholesterol more than 1.2 mmol per litre, but if you have diabetes your doctor will aim for a total cholesterol of less than 4.0 mmol per litre and LDL less than 2.0 mmol per litre.

### How can I tell if my cholesterol is high?

Very occasionally a high cholesterol level will cause yellow waxy-looking plaques in the skin around the eyes called xanthelasma, or fatty lumps on the elbows called xanthomas. But in the vast majority of cases there is no obvious outside sign that your cholesterol is high and the only way to know is to have a blood test. As someone with diabetes, your GP will want to do a blood test every year to check your cholesterol.

## How can my cholesterol be high if I eat healthily?

Only about 10–20 per cent of your total cholesterol comes from what you eat. The rest is made by your body, and that amount is genetically predetermined. That is why it is possible to find fat people who eat a high cholesterol diet but still have low cholesterol in their bloodstream, and others who eat healthily but who have high cholesterol because their bodies make more of it.

## Why does cholesterol matter?

High levels of cholesterol can cause fatty plaques to form on the walls of the blood vessels. Over time these plaques can build up and harden, forming what is known as atherosclerosis or hardening of the arteries, which can mean not enough blood being delivered to certain parts of the body. If the plaques form in the coronary arteries this causes heart disease. If they form in the blood vessels supplying the brain, they can cause strokes and if they form in the vessels in the legs, they can cause severe pain in the legs when walking. This is called claudication. Sometime blood clots form on the plaques and if they break off, they can then block an artery which means no blood can get through and this can mean a heart attack, stroke or gangrene. It is thought that high cholesterol is implicated in half of all heart attacks but, of course, cholesterol isn't the whole story. There are several other risk factors that play a role.

## Do I need treatment for my cholesterol?

Your GP will advise you to address any lifestyle issues that could increase your risk. So if you smoke, you should stop, and your doctor will be able to help you with advice about local smoking cessation services. You should aim for a healthy BMI of between 18.5

and 25 kg/m$^2$ (or 23 if you are of Asian descent; see Chapter 1 for how to calculate BMI). You should restrict your alcohol to recommended limits – that's 14 units a week for women and 21 units a week for men, with at least two dry days a week. Watch your salt and fat intake and try to keep to a low cholesterol diet. You should also aim to exercise for 30 minutes at least 5 times a week. Your GP will advise on whether you need to take medication but as someone with diabetes you are more likely to need medication.

## What does treatment involve?

The most common type of medicine used to treat high cholesterol is a group of drugs called statins. They work by inhibiting an enzyme in the liver which reduces the production of cholesterol. You will need a blood test to check your liver is healthy before starting treatment and three months later. If all is well you will just need your liver blood tests to be monitored once a year. Statins are generally well tolerated but in some people they can cause muscle aches. These are usually mild but rarely they can lead to serious muscle problems so it is important that you report any symptoms to your doctor who will probably want to do a blood test to check your muscle enzymes. If these are very raised it suggests muscle damage and your doctor will advise that you stop your statin.

There is also a drug called ezetimibe, which works by blocking absorption of cholesterol from the gut. By definition this could only ever reduce your total cholesterol by a maximum of 20 per cent but it is useful in patients who cannot tolerate statins or it can be used in conjunction with a statin for those with very high cholesterol levels.

# 7

# Diabetic eye disease

Diabetes can affect your eyes in several ways, which is why you will be called for eye screening every year. It is important that you go to these appointments, as they will pick up any problems early and the treatment is more likely to be effective. If you are registered with an NHS GP you will automatically be called for a screening examination every year. At this appointment you will have drops put into your eye to dilate the pupil, allowing the doctor to view the back of the eye more clearly. They will take a digital photograph to look in detail at the blood vessels at the back of the eye, but this is not the same as the routine eye test done by an optometrist so it is important that you also make your own appointment each year to have your eyes tested with an optometrist.

## Diabetic retinopathy

We know that diabetes affects the small blood vessels in the back of the eye, which can cause either blockage or leakage of the vessels. In the early stages you may not be aware of any change in your vision, but if left untreated this can cause serious visual problems and even blindness, which is why it is so important to attend your screening appointments. Forty per cent of people with type 1 diabetes and 20 per cent of people with type 2 diabetes will develop some form of retinopathy. There are two main types.

### Background retinopathy

This is the most common type of diabetic retinopathy. It may show as small bulges in the blood vessels in the back of the eye, known as microaneurysms, or as leakage of fluid or blood. As long as it doesn't involve the macula, which is the central area of the back of the eye responsible for our central vision, our colour vision and fine detail, you would not be aware that anything was wrong.

## Proliferative retinopathy

This is a more progressive form of retinopathy where the blood vessels at the back of the eye become blocked, meaning the retina cannot get its oxygen supply. The retina reacts to this by developing new blood vessels, which is called neovascularization. It sounds great, doesn't it, but the new vessels are weak and bleed easily. If there is a large bleed this may obscure vision completely in that eye. It sometimes improves if the blood is reabsorbed but repetitive bleeds can lead to scarring, which may distort the retina and can actually lead to the retina becoming detached with serious loss of vision.

## Diabetic maculopathy

The macula as I have said is the most important part of our retina when it comes to our eyesight. It can be involved in background or proliferative retinopathy. If the macula is involved, sadly, your central vision may be significantly reduced meaning you may struggle to read or recognize faces.

## How is diabetic retinopathy treated?

The whole aim of the diabetic screening is to pick up any changes early when they are most amenable to laser treatment to prevent bleeding or regrowth of new vessels. The laser treatment is sometimes directed at a specific area or more widely to a larger area. The greater the area of the retina that needs to be treated, the more likely you are to notice a change in your vision after treatment but it is important to have the treatment as not treating the lesions would ultimately lead to a worse deterioration in your vision. Laser treatment is usually an outpatient treatment. You will have drops in your eye to dilate the pupil and numb the front of the eye and, as the treatment is being done, you will be asked to look in different directions so that the specialist can target the laser at specific areas of your retina. Most patients don't find this uncomfortable, but if you need extensive laser therapy you may notice some discomfort or a headache after your treatment.

## Cataracts

Anyone can get cataracts, and many older people do, but they tend to occur earlier in people with diabetes. Cataracts occur when the normally clear lens starts to cloud over. You may notice a loss of vision and a glare, particularly at night. Cataracts can be treated by removing the opaque lens and replacing it with a clear artificial lens. This can be done under local or general anaesthetic.

## Glaucoma

Glaucoma is a condition where fluid in the eye doesn't drain properly, which can lead to a rise in pressure in the eye and ultimately, if not treated, to loss of vision. In the early stages you may not be aware of any symptoms, which is why it is important that everyone has regular eye tests. Glaucoma is more common in people with diabetes and that is another reason why eye tests are free for people with diabetes.

## What can I do to protect my vision?

It is important that you try to keep your blood sugar levels as well controlled as possible to protect your vision and you should make it a priority to attend your annual diabetic eye screening appointment and to see your optometrist every year as the two appointments look for different eye problems.

# 8

# Kidney disease

Diabetic kidney disease is also referred to as diabetic nephropathy and affects around 40 per cent of all people with diabetes. It simply refers to deterioration in kidney function, which is generally related to high blood glucose levels and/or high blood pressure.

## How would I know if I had diabetic nephropathy?

In the early stages you may have no symptoms whatsoever, which is why it is so important that you attend for regular diabetic reviews, where the doctors and nurses can check for any early signs of kidney disease by dip-stick testing your urine for the presence of protein. There are five stages of diabetic nephropathy and symptoms only usually develop in the later stages. It can take 20 years for these signs to develop and they may include:

- blood in the urine
- swollen ankles
- shortness of breath on exertion
- fatigue
- nausea and vomiting
- a grey tinge to the skin.

## What can I do to protect myself from developing diabetic nephropathy?

It can be difficult to see why doctors and nurses get so concerned about sugar and blood pressure control if you have diabetes, but there is good evidence that if we can achieve good blood sugar control we can reduce the incidence of diabetic kidney disease significantly. So, it may be tiresome, but taking your diabetes seriously will really help.

## How is diabetic nephropathy treated?

How your condition is treated will depend on a number of factors –
how advanced the disease is, how well you are, and your own wishes.
In the early stages it is a case of eating healthily and exercising
regularly, not smoking, keeping your blood pressure under control
and monitoring your blood glucose levels closely. If the disease pro-
gresses you may need dialysis or even transplantation.

# 9

# Diabetic nerve damage

Diabetes damages small blood vessels and that includes those supplying the nerves. This means that essential nutrients cannot get
to the nerves and, over many years, this causes damage to the
nerves known as neuropathy. There are three different types of
neuropathy.

## Sensory neuropathy

This involves damage to the nerves of sensation, which relay feel-
ings of touch, pain, temperature and an awareness of where your
joints are, which is called proprioception. We don't ever think
about where our joints are but if your sensory nerves are working
well you automatically know where your feet and hands are, for
example. When people with diabetes develop sensory neuropathy,
the nerves in the feet are the most commonly affected, which is
one of the reasons why people with diabetes are entitled to free
chiropody. If you can't feel pain in your feet you could easily cut
your skin when cutting your toenails and be unaware and be at risk
of infection. It really is worth seeing a chiropodist regularly if you
have diabetes as you could have an ulcer on your foot from fric-
tion or even a stone in your shoe that you are unaware of. If left
untreated that could grow or become infected and be much more
difficult to treat.

## Autonomic neuropathy

Your autonomic nervous system is the nerves that automatically
carry messages between your organs and your brain. They are
responsible for things like bowel movements, bladder control, heart
rate and sweating. If these nerves become damaged then you may
develop difficulties with bladder or bowel control, rapid heart rate
or spontaneous sweating.

## Motor neuropathy

If your diabetes affects the nerves that control your muscles you may develop muscle weakness, cramps or involuntary twitching in your muscles.

## How is neuropathy treated?

Good blood glucose control can reduce the progression of neuropathy and your doctor will be able to help with medication to target some of the symptoms associated with neuropathy depending on which nerves are affected.

## How can I prevent neuropathy?

The single most important thing that you can do is to try to maintain good glucose control. It is also important that you attend for regular review with your diabetes nurse and have your feet checked at least once a year.

# 10

# Sexual problems

I have talked at length about the problems with nerve and blood vessel damage associated with diabetes and, unfortunately, the nerves and vessels supplying the sex organs can also be affected. This can lead to erectile dysfunction in men and vaginal dryness and loss of sensation in women. People with diabetes are also often on a cocktail of prescription medicines that may affect sexual desire or function, so if you are concerned, please don't stop your medication but do talk to your doctor who may be able to offer you an alternative.

## Thrush

One other condition that I really feel I ought to mention here is thrush. It is not uncommon to pick up previously undiagnosed diabetes because the person has been plagued with recurrent thrush. This is because the fungus that causes thrush thrives on high-sugar levels. Thrush is caused by a yeast called *Candida albicans*, which is actually present in the vagina of 20 per cent of women without causing symptoms. If it does cause symptoms, it is likely to cause soreness and itching in the vagina and vulva and a cottage cheese-like discharge.

### Who gets thrush?

Thrush is extremely common. Poorly controlled (or undiagnosed) diabetes can be a cause but it is also more common in the following instances.

- *Pregnancy* Hormonal changes in pregnancy can increase the likelihood of developing thrush.
- *Antibiotics* It is normal for vaginas to contain bacteria and, when in the right balance, these bacteria play a role in keeping the vagina clean and healthy. If you have antibiotics for an infection

elsewhere in the body, that can reduce the amount of bacteria in your vagina meaning that the yeast that causes thrush can proliferate to cause symptoms.

- *Steroids* Taking steroids increases the likelihood of developing thrush.
- *Immune problems* AIDS or taking drugs to damp down your immune system for other conditions you may have, can make you more prone to thrush.

Contrary to popular belief, taking the combined oral contraceptive pill has not been proven to make you more prone to thrush but if I see a woman with recurrent thrush who is using the combined pill, I sometimes suggest an alternative form of contraception and occasionally it does the trick.

## Will I have to have a swab test?

I don't always swab women with symptoms of thrush. If you have had it before, recognize the symptoms and are in a monogamous relationship, you may simply need the treatment, which can come in the form of creams, pessaries or tablets. If, however, there is any possibility of a sexually transmitted infection your doctor will want to check this out with a swab test.

## What can I do to prevent thrush developing?

If you suffer with recurrent thrush, make sure you only use underwear made with natural fibres. Avoid man-made fibres, which are likely to make you sweat, and, wherever possible, keep clothing loose. Try to avoid any perfumed products as this will alter the naturally acidic environment of the vagina and mean that the yeast can thrive. The yeast that causes thrush grows in the bowel so after going to the toilet always wipe front to back to avoid encouraging the yeast forward to the vaginal opening. Thrush is not a sexually transmitted infection but some women notice flares after sexual intercourse – if this is you, make sure you use plenty of lubricant during sex to reduce any trauma to the delicate vaginal skin. I often recommend a daily probiotic to maintain good gut health and keep the yeast in balance too. If you suffer with recurrent thrush your doctor may suggest a longer course of treatment.

# 11

# Diabetes and pregnancy

Pregnancy can cause sugar levels to rise, meaning some women who did not have diabetes before develop diabetes in pregnancy. This is called gestational diabetes and should resolve after the baby is born, but it is associated with an increased risk of developing type 2 diabetes later in life. Having diabetes shouldn't put you off having a baby but you do need to be aware of the possible risks and be prepared to keep a close eye on your blood sugar levels as good glucose control undoubtedly reduces the risks. In an ideal world, if you know you have diabetes, it is better to plan your pregnancy as good preconception care will also help. Pregnant women with diabetes have an increased risk of:

- miscarriage
- larger babies
- premature births
- pre-eclampsia
- blood clots
- caesarean section
- stillbirth.

Babies born to mothers with diabetes have an increased risk of:

- being born with congenital abnormalities
- respiratory distress at birth
- low blood sugar at birth
- jaundice.

This list must look very frightening, I know, and I don't want to scare you. With good antenatal and perinatal care there is every chance of you being a healthy mum and having a healthy baby. I have lots of patients with diabetes who have happy, healthy families but it is a time when you need to take your diabetic care extra seriously in order to achieve the best outcome for all.

# 12

# Travelling with diabetes

There is no reason why you shouldn't travel wherever you like if you have diabetes but you will have to give a little more thought to your travelling than most.

## Before you travel

Along with all the holiday vaccinations that everyone else has to plan, you will have to make sure that you have plenty of medication to cover your holiday. If your repeat prescription is likely to run out your GP will happily issue your next prescription early and if you need to use needles for insulin, ask your tour operator if you need a covering letter from your GP. Make sure you have a free European Health Insurance Card (EHIC) if you are travelling in Europe and health insurance if you are travelling elsewhere.

## Packing for your holiday

Take a list of all your medications with you so that if you should lose any, you can tell a local doctor exactly what you are on. You will need to take both the brand name and the generic name as drugs have different brand names in different countries. Pack extra medication in your hand luggage in case of delays and, similarly, take extra snacks with you as you may not be in control of when you eat your meals. Think ahead with time zones so that you can plan your medication times appropriately.

If you are on insulin you will need to carry that with you in hand luggage, as it could be affected by the temperatures in the hold. Alternatively, you could store it in a flask in your main luggage but make sure that you check it when you arrive at your destination. If it has crystals in it, it has been affected by the temperature and you should replace it.

# 13

## Recipes

### Starters and light meals

#### Lemon tuna pâté with sweetcorn and horseradish

*Prep* 15 mins. *Serves* 4

Pâté can often be made with rich ingredients that, although tasty, can be high in saturated fats. Try this healthier version instead – the tuna is brought to life with a combination of lemon and horseradish, giving this appetizer a delicious kick of flavour. Vegetables aren't typically added to pâté, but here the sweetcorn brings interesting texture as well as fibre. You can experiment by adding finely diced red peppers too. Serve with lightly toasted sourdough or rye bread. If you prefer a rougher texture or don't have a food processor, simply mash the tuna with a fork.

*170 g / 6 oz / 1 cup canned, flaked tuna, drained*

*55 g / 2 oz / ¼ cup half-fat spread*

*10 ml / 2 tsps horseradish sauce, or to taste*

*10 ml / 2 tsps lemon juice, or to taste*

*100 g / 3½ oz / ½ cup canned sweetcorn kernels*

***To garnish:***
*Wafer-thin slices of cucumber with skin left on*

Put the tuna and half-fat spread into a food processor or blender and whizz until smooth (or mash with a fork). Add the horseradish and lemon juice to taste, mix well and stir in the sweetcorn. Spoon into ramekins and garnish with the thinly sliced cucumber.

## Summer pea soup with bacon

This vibrant soup is simple to make, and can be served hot or chilled. Although fresh peas will impart a better flavour, it works just as well with frozen peas, which can often give a brighter colour than fresh. Choose lean bacon to keep the saturated fat content down. No need to add salt as there's plenty in the bacon.

*Prep* 5 mins. *Cook* 20 mins. *Serves* 4

1 small onion, finely chopped

570 ml / 20 fl oz / 2½ cups chicken stock

285 g / 10 oz / 2 cups fresh or frozen peas

285 ml / 10 fl oz / 1⅓ cups skimmed or semi-skimmed milk

45 g / 1½ oz / ¼ cup diced lean bacon

White pepper, to taste

**To garnish:**

45 ml / 1½ oz / 3 tbsps
0 per cent fat Greek yogurt

A few freshly chopped chives

Simmer the onion in the chicken stock for about 5 mins or until softened. Add the peas and simmer for a further 5 mins. Add the milk and transfer to a blender or food processor and whizz for a couple of mins until smooth. Strain or sieve back into the pan, add the bacon and cook for a further 3–4 mins, then season to taste. Serve each portion garnished with a swirl of Greek yogurt and a scattering of freshly chopped chives.

## Tomato soup with basil

This is a bit of a cheat's recipe as it uses passata (sieved tomatoes) so there's no need to spend time skinning, de-seeding, chopping and sieving fresh tomatoes. Passata is widely available in supermarkets and should be a staple in any (cheating) cook's cupboard. The sugar in the recipe is not essential – it's only a teaspoon between 4 servings but that is just enough to counteract the acidity in the tomatoes. If you like, you could add a little freshly chopped garlic to the stock. For a vegetarian option, use vegetable rather than chicken stock.

*Prep* 3 mins. *Cook* 10 mins. *Serves* 4

*570 ml / 1pint / 2½ cups passata*

*285 ml / 10 fl oz / 1⅛ cups chicken stock (from half a cube)*

*10 ml / 1 dessertspoon red pesto*

*Few basil leaves, torn*

*5 ml / 1 tsp sugar*

*Pinch of salt and freshly ground black pepper, to taste*

**For the croutons:**
*Two 45 g / 1½ oz slices granary or seeded bread, crusts removed*

**To garnish:**
*45 ml / 1½ oz / 3 tbsps low-fat Greek yogurt*

*4 small sprigs fresh basil*

Put the passata and chicken stock into a pan and bring to the boil. Add the pesto, basil leaves and sugar. Season to taste. Lower heat and simmer for 5 mins. Meanwhile, toast the bread on both sides and dice into crouton shapes. Serve each portion with a swirl of yogurt and garnished with a sprig of fresh basil. Serve the croutons separately so they stay crunchy.

## Artichoke, mushroom and cherry tomato salad

This is a light starter that is ideal for *al fresco* dining. If you want to make it more substantial for a light lunch, add salad leaves, lightly steamed fine green beans, and baby new potatoes boiled in their skins. The addition of olive oil helps to reduce the sharpness of the French dressing but you can omit it if you like.

*Prep* 10 mins. *Serves* 4

*340 g / 12 oz / 2½ cups canned artichoke hearts, drained*

*115 g / 4 oz button mushrooms, wiped and halved*

*170 g / 6 oz cherry tomatoes*

*60 ml / 4 tbsps oil-free French dressing*

*10 ml / 2 tsps extra-virgin olive oil*

**To garnish:**
*A sprinkling of your favourite herbs, chopped, e.g. chives, parsley, thyme*

Combine the artichoke hearts, mushrooms and cherry tomatoes in a bowl. Mix the French dressing with the olive oil in a bottle or screw-top jar, shaking vigorously. Pour over the salad and mix well. Transfer to four individual plates or small bowls before serving, garnished with freshly chopped herbs.

## Lebanese tabbouleh salad

This brightly coloured salad is equally good when served as a supper, starter or a light snack. It's packed with flavour and is very simple to prepare. Traditionally it doesn't contain red and yellow peppers, but it's a good idea to get into the habit of adding extra veg to your recipes for good health. Choose fine or coarse bulgur wheat according to your taste – note that the coarser type may take a few more mins to cook.

*Prep* 20 mins. *Serves* 4

*200 g / 7 oz / 1 heaped cup fine bulgur wheat*

*55 g / 2 oz / ½ cup spring onions, finely chopped*

*115 g / 4 oz / 1 cup green pepper, diced*

*115 g / 4 oz / 1 cup yellow pepper, diced*

*170 g / 6 oz cherry tomatoes, left whole*

*60 g / 2 oz / 1 cup fresh parsley, finely chopped*

*30 ml / 2 tbsps fresh coriander, finely chopped*

*45 ml / 3 tbsps lemon juice*

*15 ml / 1 tbsp extra-virgin olive oil*

*Pinch of salt and freshly ground black pepper, to taste*

Put the bulgur wheat into a large bowl, cover with boiling water and leave to soak for 15 mins. In the meantime, prepare the vegetables. Transfer the bulgur wheat to a sieve, pressing down on it to remove any remaining liquid – it should be as dry as you can get it. Turn into a serving bowl and mix with the spring onions, peppers, cherry tomatoes and herbs. Mix the lemon juice with the olive oil, season to taste and toss through the bulgur wheat mixture before serving. Serve chilled.

## Olive tapenade bruschetta

Tapenade is an olive purée that has a distinctive flavour and is used to liven up fish, pasta or vegetables. It's delicious simply served with tomatoes on crusty bread. You'll find it in jars from most super-markets and it's a really useful addition to your store cupboard for those quick and easy meal ideas. You could also top this bruschetta with roasted peppers, artichokes, anchovies, capers or even chunky halved olives – a summer favourite that will transport you back to the shores of the Mediterranean.

*Prep* 10 mins. *Serves* 4

*15 ml / 1 tbsp olive oil*

*2 cloves garlic, crushed*

*365 g / 13 oz / 2 cups ripe tomatoes, sliced*

*4–5 sprigs basil, torn*

*Freshly ground black pepper*

*1 crusty granary or wholemeal loaf (approx. 140 g / 5 oz), cut into 8 slices*

*10 g / 2 tsps olive tapenade*

Mix together the olive oil and crushed garlic and pour over the sliced tomatoes. Add in the torn basil leaves and season with pepper. Grill the crusty slices of bread until golden and spread with the tapenade. Top with the flavoured tomato slices and serve immediately.

## Nutty prawns

Peanut butter, be it smooth or crunchy, has a similar type of fibre, soluble fibre, to that found in beans and lentils and it is an integral part of healthy eating. Peanut butter also contains a range of vitamins including vitamin E and the B vitamins. This versatile and universal cholesterol-free marinade works a treat with any tiger prawns, tofu, chunks of meat, in fact anything that needs sprucing up! You can use it immediately, for example, to coat chicken wings before cooking, or you can use it to marinade a whole roast in the fridge for up to 24 hours. These prawns are simply brushed with the nutty marinade and then stir-fried. Alternatively, cook on a barbecue or under a hot grill.

*Prep* 5 mins. *Cook* 5–10 mins. *Serves* 4

*280 g / 10 oz / 1½ cups tiger prawns, shelled and ready to cook*

**For the marinade:**

*2.5-cm / 1-inch piece root ginger, grated*

*2 cloves garlic, crushed*

*1 tbsp / 15 ml groundnut (peanut) oil*

*1 tbsp / 15 ml honey*

*2 tsps / 10 ml coarse grain mustard*

*70 g / 2½ oz / 4 tbsp crunchy or smooth peanut butter*

*2 tbsps / 30 ml light soy sauce*

*15 g / ½ oz coriander leaves, finely chopped*

*75 ml / 5 tbsps cold water*

*70 g / 2½ oz / 4 tbsps crunchy or smooth peanut butter*

*2 tbsps / 30 ml light soy sauce*

Mix all the marinade ingredients together and brush over the prawns. Stir-fry in a non-stick pan until prawns are cooked but still juicy; add a little hot water if necessary and serve immediately.

## Grilled feta cheese and red peppers

This starter is a party in your mouth – a burst of creamy yet crumbly feta cheese, interspersed with crunchy bits of fresh red peppers, and a tang of citrus. Serve as a light meal with some warm wholemeal pitta bread or tortilla wrap.

*Prep* 5 mins. *Cook* 5 mins. *Serves* 2

115 g / 4 oz feta cheese

5 ml / 1 tsp ground cumin

1 head of lettuce, torn

1 red pepper, diced

10 ml / 2 tbsps fat-free French dressing

1 fresh orange

15 g / ½ oz fresh coriander, roughly chopped

Preheat the grill to medium and line a grill pan with foil. Cut the feta into eight slices and lay these on the foil. Sprinkle on the ground cumin and grill, one side only, until the cheese starts to brown. Lay the torn lettuce leaves, coriander leaves and the red peppers on to a plate and drizzle on the dressing. Cut the orange in half: squeeze one half on to the dressed salad and cut the other half into wedges. Serve the feta cheese on top of the dressed salad leaves. Garnish with orange wedges.

# Main meals

## Lamb steaks with potato ratatouille

The idea of combining lamb with ratatouille that contains potatoes may sound strange, but with this recipe you get your protein, veg and carbs all in one go, so there's no need for extra accompaniments. You'll find that this particular ratatouille mix marries well with chicken or turkey. New boiled potatoes in their skins are easy to use as there's no peeling or chopping, and the added bonus is that they're likely to have a more favourable effect on your blood glucose than large potatoes without the skins.

*Prep* 10 mins. *Cook* 25 mins. *Serves* 4

285 g / 10 oz / 2 cups new baby potatoes, unpeeled and halved if desired

15 ml / 1 tbsp olive oil

115 g / 4 oz / 1 cup onions, finely chopped

1 garlic clove, crushed

225 g / 8 oz / 2 cups courgettes, sliced

115 g / 4 oz / 1 cup baby aubergine, diced

455 g / 1lb / 2 cups canned or fresh tomatoes, chopped

60 ml / 2 fl oz / ¼ cup white wine

5 ml / ⅛ oz / 1 tsp caster sugar

Good pinch dried herbes de Provence (Mediterranean mixed herbs)

4 lean lamb steaks cut from the leg (approx. 115 g / 4 oz each)

Pinch of salt and freshly ground black pepper, to taste

4 small sprigs fresh rosemary

Put the potatoes in a pan of salted water, bring to the boil and parboil for 5 mins. Meanwhile, heat the olive oil in a large non-stick pan, and gently sauté the onion and garlic for 2–3 mins until soft but not browned. Add the rest of the vegetables, including the tomatoes, white wine, sugar and herbs and gently bring to a boil. When the potatoes are parboiled, drain them and tip them into the pan along with the rest of the vegetables. Lower the heat, and let the mixture simmer for 5–10 mins until the vegetables are cooked, stirring occasionally. Meanwhile, cook the lamb steaks under a medium grill for 5–6 mins each side, or until done as you like them. Season the ratatouille to taste, and serve with the lamb steaks, garnished with sprigs of fresh rosemary.

## Lamb cutlets with tomato and mint sauce

This sauce is refreshing and light and helps to balance the richness of lamb. The dish is delicious served with mashed potatoes to soak up the sauce and a medley of green vegetables such as wilted spinach and fine green beans.

*Prep* 5 mins. *Cook* 15 mins. *Serves* 4

*4 lean lamb escalopes (approx. 100 g / 3½ oz each)*

*Good pinch dried rosemary*

*Freshly ground black pepper*

*2 tsps balsamic vinegar*

**Tomato and mint sauce:**

*700 g / 1¾ lbs / 3½ cups cherry tomatoes, halved*

*10 leaves of fresh mint (or 1 tsp mint sauce)*

*1–2 tsps lemon juice*

*Freshly ground black pepper*

Preheat the grill to medium. To make the sauce: In a shallow open pan, place the tomato halves with 30 ml / 2 tbsps of water and the mint leaves and simmer for about 10 mins until soft. Add the lemon juice (and mint sauce, if using) and then liquidize until smooth. Season and reheat. Meanwhile flavour the lamb cutlets with rosemary, pepper and balsamic vinegar and grill under a medium heat until cooked (approx. 5 mins each side or as desired) and serve with the sauce.

## Warm chicken salad

A main-course salad that would also serve six as a starter. Use brightly coloured salad leaves to add interest and variety of flavour. The salad dressing can be made in advance and kept in the fridge until needed. Try serving with noodles, or accompany with toasted wholemeal pitta bread strips.

*Prep* 5 mins. *Cook* 10 mins. *Serves* 4

*15 g / ½ oz / 1 tbsp plain flour*

*Good pinch black pepper*

*Fresh lemon thyme sprigs*

*400 g / 14 oz / 1½ cups chicken breast fillets, cut into bite-sized pieces*

*110 g / 4 oz / 1 cup mangetout*

*15 ml / 1 tbsp olive oil*

*140 g / 5 oz / 1 cup cherry tomatoes, halved*

*85 g / 3 oz / 1 cup mixed salad leaves*

*30 g / 1 oz / ¼ cup spring onions, chopped*

**To garnish:**
*5 g / ¼ oz / 1 tsp chives, finely chopped*

*A large pinch of sesame seeds*

**For the salad dressing:**
*15 ml / 1 tbsp balsamic vinegar*

*15 ml / 1 tbsp sesame seed oil*

*15 ml / 1 tbsp soy sauce*

*30 g / 1 oz / ¼ cup spring onions, chopped*

Mix the flour with the pepper and lemon thyme and coat the chicken breast pieces with this seasoned flour. Steam the mangetout over a little boiling water for 1–2 mins. then drain. Make the dressing by mixing all the ingredients together. Heat the olive oil and cook the chicken pieces for 5 mins, turning once. Add the steamed mangetout and cherry tomatoes and cook for a further 1–2 mins. Arrange the salad leaves and chopped spring onions on a serving plate. Pile the warm chicken and vegetable mixture on top of the salad and drizzle over the dressing. Sprinkle with the chives and sesame seeds before serving.

## Cold chicken with red pepper sauce

An alternative to creamy sauces or mayonnaise, this red pepper sauce is delightfully light and low in calories. It could also be made with yellow peppers and a ribbon of red and yellow peppers could be spooned over the chicken to give contrasting colours. If you fancy converting this into a chilled soup, simply add a little extra yogurt to the sauce to thin it down, finely shred the chicken and mix with the pepper sauce, pop it in the fridge and top with fresh basil leaves before serving.

*Prep* 10 mins. *Serves* 4

*2 red peppers (approx. 170 g / 6 oz each)*

*1 clove garlic, chopped*

*15 ml / 3 tsps dry sherry*

*425 g / 15 oz / 2 cups low-fat natural yogurt*

**Serve with**:
*4 grilled chicken breasts (approx. 110 g / 4 oz each) seasoned with a pinch of salt and freshly ground black pepper, to taste*

**To garnish**:
*Watercress*

Remove the skins from the red peppers by blackening the peppers over a flame and then scraping the skin off. Remove the stalks and take the seeds out. Chop the peppers finely and place in a blender with the chopped garlic and the sherry. Blend until smooth and then mix in the yogurt. Serve chilled with cold grilled chicken and garnish with watercress.

## Pork with fresh plums

Plums make a great low-fat base for this delicious, pink sauce, and keeping their skins on helps to preserve the fibre content. The shredded cabbage adds crunch and texture. All you need for a complete meal is to serve this with steamed brown basmati rice.

*Prep* 5 mins. *Cook* 25 mins. *Serves* 4

*500 g / 18 oz / 3 cups fresh plums, stoned and halved*

*170 g / 6 oz / 3 cups white cabbage, finely shredded*

*285 ml / 10 fl. oz / 1⅓ cups chicken stock*

*400 g / 14 oz / 2 cups lean pork fillet, cut into bite-sized pieces*

*10 ml / 2 tsps rapeseed oil*

*Freshly ground black pepper*

*1 large onion (225 g / 8 oz / 2 cups), finely sliced*

*Freshly ground black pepper*

Simmer the plums in chicken stock for 5 mins. Remove and purée the plums (including the skins) and stock. In a large frying pan, heat the oil and cook the onion until soft. Add the raw shredded cabbage and continue to cook for a further 3 mins. Add the pork pieces to brown and then the puréed plums. Season, cover and simmer for 15 mins.

## Pork steaks with creamy mustard sauce

Choose pork steaks that are lean, or trim off the excess fat. The mustard enhances the flavour. Serve with a crisp green salad and seeded bread, or some lightly cooked vegetables.

*Prep* 5 mins. *Cook* 15 mins. *Serves* 4

10 ml / 2 tsps rapeseed oil

4 lean pork steaks (approx. 112 g / 4 oz each), trimmed of any fat

1 onion (approx. 84 g / 3 oz / ⅔ cup), finely chopped

140 ml / 5 fl. oz / ⅔ cup chicken stock, hot

168 g / 6 oz / ⅔ cup low-fat natural yogurt

20 g / 2 dessertspoons wholegrain mustard

Heat a heavy-based frying pan or griddle, add the oil and pan fry the pork steaks for about 10 mins. Remove from the pan and keep hot, ready for serving. To the residue in the frying pan, add the onion and cook until soft. Add the hot stock and cook for another 5 mins. Remove from the heat and stir in the yogurt and mustard. Gently reheat a little, stirring continuously to prevent the yogurt from curdling, and serve poured over the pork steaks.

## Turkey koftas

These sausage-like kebabs can be served in a variety of ways. Try them with saffron-infused basmati rice and grilled vegetables; or alternatively fill some warm wholemeal pitta bread with salad, place the turkey koftas on top and drizzle with natural yogurt flavoured with mint leaves. If you have time, marinade the turkey mince for up to two hours – the koftas will taste even more exciting.

*Prep* 10 mins. *Cook* 15 mins. *Serves* 4

*340 g / 12 oz / 1½ cups turkey breast, minced*

*28 g / 1 oz / ⅔ cup fresh chopped herbs (coriander and parsley are a good combination)*

*2 cloves garlic, crushed*

*1 tsp grated fresh ginger*

*1 green chilli, finely chopped, deseeded if desired*

*Juice of ½ lemon*

*Pinch of salt and freshly ground black pepper, to taste*

*5 ml / 1 tsp olive oil*

Preheat the grill to medium. In a large bowl, combine all the ingredients except the oil and mix well with your hands. Divide the mixture into four and roll into sausages, approximately 2 cm in diameter. Guide a metal skewer through each kofta and place on a grill pan. Brush with olive oil and grill until cooked (approx. 15 mins).

## Peppery beef strips on croutons

This dish is a delight for the taste buds. All you need is a variety of lightly cooked vegetables and some good company. The pepper sauce itself is not hot, but do watch out when you bite down on the peppercorns! Serving the meat and sauce on top of a large, crunchy crouton gives a great texture and makes sure that you don't waste any of the delicious sauce.

*Prep* 5 mins. *Cook* 20 mins. *Serves* 4

4 small rounds of bread, cut from a French stick (approx. 112 g / 4 oz each)

5 ml / 1 tsp olive oil

5 ml / 1 tsp sunflower oil

1 onion (approx. 84 g / 3 oz / ⅔ cup), finely sliced

336 g / 12 oz / 1½ cups lean sirloin steak, trimmed and cut into strips

285 ml / ½ pint / 1⅓ cups beef stock, hot

168 g / 6 oz / ⅔ cup 0 per cent fat Greek yogurt

4 tsps (pink) peppercorns in brine, drained

**To garnish:**

Chopped fresh parsley

Preheat the oven to high (gas mark 7 / 220°C / 425°F). Brush the bread rounds on both sides with the olive oil and place on an oven-proof tray. Cook in the oven for 10 mins until crispy (make sure they don't burn). In a heavy-based frying pan, heat the sunflower oil and cooked the sliced onion until soft. Add the beef strips and cook for 3 mins. Remove the onion and beef from the pan and keep hot. Add the stock to the frying pan and add the peppercorns. Simmer for 5 mins, then add the beef and onion mixture and heat through. Lower the heat, stir in the yogurt and warm through being careful not to let it boil, as it will curdle. To serve, place the large bread croutons on plates and pile the beef strips in pepper sauce on top. Garnish with chopped parsley.

## Meatloaf discs

Cooking these rounds of meatloaf individually means that there's no squabbling at the dinner table about who gets the biggest slice. It also saves on cooking time. However, if you prefer, you can cook the whole mixture in a small loaf tin for about 45 mins and serve sliced. Enjoy hot or cold with potatoes and salad. Any leftover meatloaf makes a perfect sandwich filling.

*Prep* 5 mins. *Cook* 30 mins. *Serves* 4

*400 g / 14 oz / 1¾ cups lean minced beef*

*60 g / 2 oz / ½ cup onion, finely diced*

*60 g / 2 oz / ⅔ cup mushrooms, finely diced*

*2 tbsps chopped fresh herbs (e.g. chives and parsley)*

*1 egg white*

*2 tbsps Worcestershire sauce*

*2 tsps chilli sauce, optional*

*Pinch of salt and freshly ground black pepper, to taste*

*2 tsps sunflower seeds*

*2 tbsps Worcestershire sauce*

Preheat the oven to gas mark 5 / 190°C / 375°F. In a large bowl, mix together all the ingredients, except the seeds, with your hands. Divide the mixture into quarters and press into a Yorkshire pudding tray or individual tartlet tray. Scatter with sunflower seeds. Cover with tinfoil and bake for about 20 mins until cooked.

## Parchment-baked cod

If serving this dish at a dinner party, simply put the fish parcel on a plate and allow your guests to open it up and release the citrus aroma. Lemon and spring onions delicately flavour this fish but do not overpower it. Serve it simply, with new potatoes in their skins and steamed vegetables.

*Prep 5* mins. *Cook* 20 mins. *Serves* 4

Greaseproof (parchment) paper

500 g / 4 chunks of cod fillets, skinned

30 g / 1 oz / ¼ cup spring onions, chopped

1 lemon, juice and rind

Pinch of salt and freshly ground black pepper, to taste

Preheat the oven to gas mark 6 / 200°C / 400°F. Cut four pieces of greaseproof paper, each approximately 30 cm square. On each square place a fillet of cod, some spring onions, lemon rind and juice. Season to taste. Make the greaseproof paper into parcels, sealing all the edges by using double folds. Place each on a large baking tray and bake for 20 mins before serving.

## Tuna and sweetcorn tagliatelle

Canned sweetcorn is quick and convenient, but if you fancy a fresher taste, you could cook two corn on the cobs in boiling water for 10 mins and then use the kernels scraped from the cobs. Some sweet red peppers are a colourful addition. The yogurt gives a creamy flavour and a clever way to stop it curdling is to add some cornflour.

*Prep* 5 mins. *Cook* 15 mins. *Serves* 4

300 g / 10½ oz / 3½ cups dried tagliatelle

15 ml olive oil

1 large clove garlic, crushed

Red pepper, sliced

Yellow pepper, sliced

140 g / 5 oz / ⅔ cup low-fat Greek yogurt, blended with 1 tsp cornflour

280 g / 10 oz / 1½ cups canned tuna in brine, drained

1 large can (400 g) sweetcorn in water, drained

Freshly ground black pepper

2 tbsps chopped parsley

Cook the tagliatelle in boiling salted water until *al dente* (normally about 10–12 mins) and then drain. Heat the olive oil in a large pan and add the crushed garlic with the sliced peppers. Lower the heat and stir in the yogurt. Mix in the cooked tagliatelle and then add the drained tuna and sweetcorn. Stir well to combine all the ingredients and heat gently. Add some freshly ground black pepper to taste and sprinkle with chopped parsley, before turning out on to warmed serving plates.

## Pilchard pastries

Canned pilchards and sardines are economical and convenient ways to get your omega-3 fats. This recipe can use either – mixing them with mushrooms and cheese makes the dish less 'fishy'. Buy ready-made filo pastry, which is easy to use and is lower in fat and calories than regular pastry. Most recipes using filo call for oil in between the layers, which means your dish could end up being just as calorific as other pastry! Try skimmed milk or beaten egg instead. Remember to keep the filo pastry damp until you need it – try covering it with a damp kitchen towel.

*Prep* 15 mins. *Cook* 30 mins. *Serves* 4

110 g / 4 oz / 1 cup onion, finely chopped

85 g / 3 oz / 1 cup mushrooms, finely chopped

15 ml / 1 tbsp sunflower oil

425 g can (15 oz / 2½ cups) pilchards in tomato sauce

60 g / 2 oz / ⅓ cup ricotta cheese

Handful of fresh coriander leaves and stems, roughly chopped

8 sheets filo pastry (approx. 12 by 20 cm each)

30 ml / 1 fl oz skimmed milk

**To garnish:**

Lemon wedges

Fresh parsley, chopped

Preheat the oven to gas mark 5 / 190 °C / 375 °F. In a heavy-based frying pan, fry the chopped onion and mushrooms in 10 ml / 1 dessertspoon of sunflower oil until soft. Mix in the pilchards, ricotta cheese and fresh coriander leaves and stems. Take a sheet of filo pastry and brush with a little skimmed milk. Place another sheet on top. Gently lay one quarter of the fish mixture in one corner. Fold the filo pastry around the mixture, making a large triangle and sealing all the pastry joins with water. Place on a baking tray and repeat the process for the other three triangles. Brush with skimmed milk and bake for 10 mins. Remove and brush with the remaining 5 ml / 1 tsp of oil and bake for a further 5–10 mins until brown. Serve garnished with lemon wedges and parsley.

## Swordfish kebabs

Swordfish is a chunky meaty fish that works really well on skewers as it doesn't flake as easily as other fish. Cooks in minutes – treat yourself to these kebabs as part of a meat-free summer barbecue, or simply cook under a hot grill. You can use red pepper chunks instead of the water chestnuts if you prefer. Tastes great with a fresh salad jewelled with pomegranate seeds.

*Prep* 15 mins. *Cook* 15 mins. *Serves* 4

*70 g / 2½ oz fresh baby corn*

*400 g / 14 oz swordfish steaks, boned, skinned and cut into 1 cm / 1½ cm cubes*

*1 red pepper (220 g / 8 oz / 2 cups), deseeded and cut into cubes*

*220 g can (8 oz / 2 cups) water chestnuts in water, drained and cut in halves*

**Basting sauce:**

*30 ml / 2 tbsps soy sauce*

*5 ml / 1 tsp rice wine vinegar*

*Juice of 1 lemon*

*2 tsps sesame oil*

*½ tsp sugar*

Cook the baby corn in boiling water for a couple of mins until just tender. Preheat the grill to high. Mix all the ingredients for the basting sauce together in a small dish. Thread the swordfish, red pepper pieces, water chestnuts and baby corn on to four skewers. Place on a large grill pan and baste thoroughly, turning to ensure they are coated on all sides. If there are any extra vegetables, put these on the grill pan too and baste with the sauce. Place under a hot grill for 10–15 mins, ensuring that you turn the kebabs frequently so each side is fully cooked.

## Chunky hummus topped with grilled vegetables

Chick peas are so underrated! You can enjoy them cold in salads, hot in soups and curries and they're a great timesaver when you don't have any veg to hand. They're a source of protein and soluble fibre (the type that can help to reduce your blood cholesterol levels as part of a heart healthy diet), and pulses count once a day towards your 'five a day' target of fruit and vegetables. This homemade hummus becomes a main meal when it's topped with flavoursome grilled Mediterranean vegetables. Serve with warm pitta bread strips either as a starter or a lunchtime treat.

*Prep* 15 mins. *Cook* 10 mins. *Serves* 4

### Hummus:

1 can (410 g / 14 oz / 1 ½ cups) chick peas in water, drained (but reserve liquid)

2 cloves garlic, peeled

Juice of 2 lemons

60 g / 2 oz / 4 tbsps tahini (sesame seed paste)

1 red pepper, stalk and seeds removed and cut into quarters

1 yellow / orange pepper, stalk and seeds removed and cut into quarters

Pinch of salt and freshly ground black pepper, to taste

5 ml / 1 tsp olive oil

### Grilled vegetables:

110 g / 4 oz / 1 cup aubergine, thinly sliced

110 g / 4 oz / 1 cup courgette, thinly sliced

### To serve:

10 ml / 2 tsps olive oil

Paprika, for sprinkling

Preheat the grill. Make the hummus by lightly blending all the ingredients together with approximately 60 ml drained chick pea liquor in a liquidizer. Do not make it too smooth! Chill in the refrigerator. Meanwhile, lay the vegetables on a large baking tray, season and brush with the olive oil. Cook under a hot grill for 10 mins, turning once. To serve, place a mound of hummus on a large dinner plate and lay the grilled vegetables over the top. Drizzle with the olive oil and sprinkle with a little paprika.

## Fruity lentils and vegetables with cheese

This is a vibrant combination of flavours and colours – orange carrot ribbons, green pepper cubes, diced tomatoes, and apple – and to top it off there's a crunchy addition of peanuts. Enjoy this dish as a topping for jacket potatoes or a filling in tortilla wraps. If you like a hint of spice, simply throw in a chopped red chilli. Do not add salt to the liquid when boiling the lentils, as this will delay the cooking process.

*Prep* 10 mins. *Cook* 15–20 mins. *Serves* 4

110 g / 4 oz / ½ cup red lentils

200 ml / 7 fl oz / ¾ cup vegetable stock

15 ml / 1 tbsp sunflower oil

140 g / 5 oz / ¾ cup carrot, grated

1 large onion (225 g / 8 oz / 2 cups), diced

1 green pepper (170 g / 6 oz / 1½ cups), diced

110 g / 4 oz / ⅔ cup tomatoes, diced

1 large cooking apple (390 g / 14 oz / 3 cups), peeled, cored and grated

2 cloves garlic, crushed

1 tbsp chopped fresh sage

30 g / 1 oz / ¼ cup raisins

60 g / 2 oz / ⅓ cup unsalted peanuts

110 g / 4 oz / ½ cup low-fat soft cheese

Simmer the red lentils in the vegetable stock until soft (approx. 10 mins), then drain. Meanwhile heat the sunflower oil in a large frying pan and add the grated carrots, onion, green pepper, tomatoes, grated apple, garlic and sage. Mix and then cook for about 10 mins. Add the cooked lentils, raisins and peanuts to the vegetables and gently stir in the low-fat soft cheese. Heat through, then serve.

## Desserts

### Hot chocolate and chestnut soufflés

If Eve had got her eye on these little mini-soufflés, I doubt she'd have bothered with the apple, for they are almost sinfully indulgent, but oh-so-delicious! They have to be served in the little pots in which they are cooked, otherwise they will collapse, but there's no reason why on a special occasion you shouldn't go the whole hog and have a scoop of reduced fat ice-cream on the side.

*Prep* 10 mins. *Cook* 15–20 mins. *Serves* 4

*55 g / 2 oz 70 per cent cocoa chocolate*

*115 g / 4 oz / 8 level tbsps unsweetened chestnut purée*

*15 ml / ½ oz / 1 tbsp caster sugar*

*1 egg yolk*

*2 egg whites, stiffly beaten*

*Butter or margarine to grease four ramekins*

Preheat the oven to gas mark 6 / 200 °C / 400 °F. Put the chocolate into a small pan with 15 ml / 1 tbsp water and heat very gently until the chocolate has completely melted. Add the chestnut purée and caster sugar and cook, stirring until the sugar has dissolved. Remove from the heat and stir in the egg yolk, mixing thoroughly. Fold in the stiffly beaten egg whites using a large metal spoon, and transfer the mixture to four lightly greased ramekins. Stand the ramekins in a roasting tin with enough hot water to come halfway up their sides, and bake in the centre of the oven for 15–20 mins until risen and set.

## Grilled pineapple meringues

When using canned pineapple slices you may wish to double up the rings to make them thicker, but if using fresh pineapple cut the slices to about 2 cm thick instead. The meringue can be piped for a more professional finish and decorated with toasted almonds if desired. Although meringue is made from eggs, it is low in fat as you only use the egg white. Other fruits could also be used, such as peaches or fresh pears, or you could try mini meringues with apricot halves.

*Prep* 5 mins. *Cook* 5 mins. *Serves* 4

*1 large egg white*

*56 g / 2 oz / ¼ cup caster sugar*

*A pinch of cornflour*

*1 can (432 g / 15 oz / 2 cups) pineapple slices in natural juice, drained*

Heat the grill to a high temperature. Make the meringue, by whisking the egg white in a dry bowl until soft peaks are formed. Add the sugar mixed with the cornflour and continue whisking until well blended. Place the drained pineapple rings on a grill tray and cook for 2 mins, turning once. Spoon meringue mixture on top of each pineapple slice and put back under the grill. Cook for approx. 1–2 mins until the meringue is golden and then serve.

# Index